REPORT DOCUMENTATION PAGE

1. AGENCY USE ONLY (Leave blank)	2. REPORT DATE May 2009	3. REPORT TYPE AND DATES COVERED Final Report January 2006–December 2007

4. TITLE AND SUBTITLE
Drug and Alcohol Testing Results 2007 Annual Report

5. FUNDING NUMBERS
VT73A1/FVN08

6. AUTHOR(S)
Mike Redington, Eve Rutyna, Nathan Grace*, and Felicity Shanahan*

7. PERFORMING ORGANIZATION NAME(S) AND ADDRESS(ES)
U.S. Department of Transportation
Research and Innovative Technology Administration
John A. Volpe National Transportation Systems Center
55 Broadway
Cambridge, MA 02142-1093

8. PERFORMING ORGANIZATION REPORT NUMBER
DOT-VNTSC-FTA-09-01

9. SPONSORING/MONITORING AGENCY NAME(S) AND ADDRESS(ES)
U.S. Department of Transportation
Federal Transit Administration
Office of Safety and Security
Washington, DC 20590

10. SPONSORING/MONITORING AGENCY REPORT NUMBER
FTA-MA-26-5562-09-1

11. SUPPLEMENTARY NOTES
*MacroSys Research and Technology
55 Broadway
Cambridge, MA 02142-1093

12a. DISTRIBUTION/AVAILABILITY STATEMENT
This document is available to the public through the National Technical Information Service, Springfield, VA 22161.

12b. DISTRIBUTION CODE

13. ABSTRACT (Maximum 200 words)

This is the 13th annual report of the results of the Federal Transit Administration's (FTA) Drug and Alcohol Testing Program. This report summarizes the reporting requirements for calendar year 2007, the requirements of the overall drug and alcohol testing program (49 CFR Part 40 and 49 CFR Part 655), the results from the data reported for 2007, and the random drug and alcohol violation rates (the percentage of persons selected for a random test who produced a positive specimen or refused to take the test) for calendar years 1995 through 2007.

This report provides a brief overview of the drug and alcohol testing requirements for both safety-sensitive employers and employees. The official random rates for 2007 are provided, as well as the official random rate trends over the last 13 years. The results of alcohol and drug tests are provided by test type, employee category, and region. The positive testing rates for drugs and alcohol are also provided for each test type, employee category, and region.

14. SUBJECT TERMS
Alcohol testing, drug testing, random testing, safety-sensitive, violation rate

15. NUMBER OF PAGES
94

16. PRICE CODE

17. SECURITY CLASSIFICATION OF REPORT Unclassified	18. SECURITY CLASSIFICATION OF THIS PAGE Unclassified	19. SECURITY CLASSIFICATION OF ABSTRACT Unclassified	20. LIMITATION OF ABSTRACT Unlimited

METRIC/ENGLISH CONVERSION FACTORS

ENGLISH TO METRIC

LENGTH (APPROXIMATE)

1 inch (in) = 2.5 centimeters (cm)
1 foot (ft) = 30 centimeters (cm)
1 yard (yd) = 0.9 meter (m)
1 mile (mi) = 1.6 kilometers (km)

AREA (APPROXIMATE)

1 square inch (sq in, in^2) = 6.5 square centimeters (cm^2)
1 square foot (sq ft, ft^2) = 0.09 square meter (m^2)
1 square yard (sq yd, yd^2) = 0.8 square meter (m^2)
1 square mile (sq mi, mi^2) = 2.6 square kilometers (km^2)
1 acre = 0.4 hectare (he) = 4,000 square meters (m^2)

MASS - WEIGHT (APPROXIMATE)

1 ounce (oz) = 28 grams (gm)
1 pound (lb) = 0.45 kilogram (kg)
1 short ton = 2,000 pounds (lb) = 0.9 tonne (t)

VOLUME (APPROXIMATE)

1 teaspoon (tsp) = 5 milliliters (ml)
1 tablespoon (tbsp) = 15 milliliters (ml)
1 fluid ounce (fl oz) = 30 milliliters (ml)
1 cup (c) = 0.24 liter (l)
1 pint (pt) = 0.47 liter (l)
1 quart (qt) = 0.96 liter (l)
1 gallon (gal) = 3.8 liters (l)
1 cubic foot (cu ft, ft^3) = 0.03 cubic meter (m^3)
1 cubic yard (cu yd, yd^3) = 0.76 cubic meter (m^3)

TEMPERATURE (EXACT)

[(x-32)(5/9)] °F = y °C

METRIC TO ENGLISH

LENGTH (APPROXIMATE)

1 millimeter (mm) = 0.04 inch (in)
1 centimeter (cm) = 0.4 inch (in)
1 meter (m) = 3.3 feet (ft)
1 meter (m) = 1.1 yards (yd)
1 kilometer (km) = 0.6 mile (mi)

AREA (APPROXIMATE)

1 square centimeter (cm^2) = 0.16 square inch (sq in, in^2)
1 square meter (m^2) = 1.2 square yards (sq yd, yd^2)
1 square kilometer (km^2) = 0.4 square mile (sq mi, mi^2)
10,000 square meters (m^2) = 1 hectare (ha) = 2.5 acres

MASS - WEIGHT (APPROXIMATE)

1 gram (gm) = 0.036 ounce (oz)
1 kilogram (kg) = 2.2 pounds (lb)
1 tonne (t) = 1,000 kilograms (kg)
= 1.1 short tons

VOLUME (APPROXIMATE)

1 milliliter (ml) = 0.03 fluid ounce (fl oz)
1 liter (l) = 2.1 pints (pt)
1 liter (l) = 1.06 quarts (qt)
1 liter (l) = 0.26 gallon (gal)

1 cubic meter (m^3) = 36 cubic feet (cu ft, ft^3)
1 cubic meter (m^3) = 1.3 cubic yards (cu yd, yd^3)

TEMPERATURE (EXACT)

[(9/5) y + 32] °C = x °F

QUICK INCH - CENTIMETER LENGTH CONVERSION

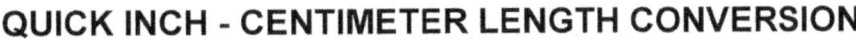
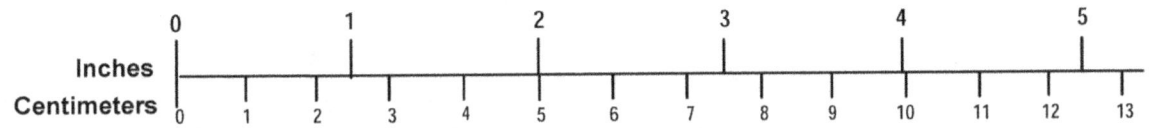

QUICK FAHRENHEIT - CELSIUS TEMPERATURE CONVERSION

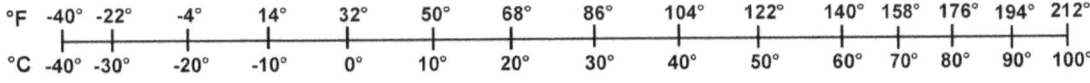

For more exact and or other conversion factors, see NIST Miscellaneous Publication 286, Units of Weights and Measures. Price $2.50 SD Catalog No. C13 10286

Updated 6/17/98

Table of Contents

Table of Contents (continued)

Table of Contents (continued)

List of Figures

List of Figures (continued)

List of Figures (continued)

List of Tables

List of Tables (continued)

List of Tables (continued)

1. Testing Requirements

1.1 Required Testing Program

Safety-sensitive employees must undergo testing for five illegal substances with the use of six different test types. Employees who perform safety-sensitive functions must also be tested for alcohol use in each of those test types, except for pre-employment testing. Employers are required to conduct four types of tests of employees who perform safety-sensitive functions and are permitted to conduct two other types of tests for drugs and alcohol (return-to-duty and follow-up).

Table 1 lists the employee categories, test types, and drug types that fall under the auspices of the FTA Drug and Alcohol Testing Program. For more detailed descriptions of each of these categories, refer to the glossary in Appendix C. You may also refer to FTA and DOT drug and alcohol regulations on the FTA Office of Safety and Security Web site at http://transit-safety.volpe.dot.gov/Safety/datesting/regulations/default.asp. For additional guidance, another excellent source is the Office of Drug and Alcohol Policy and Compliance (ODAPC) Web site http://www.dot.gov/ost/dapc/index.html.

Table 1. Safety-Sensitive Employee Categories, Test Types, and Drug Types

Safety-Sensitive Employee Categories
• Revenue Vehicle Operation
• Revenue Vehicle and Equipment Maintenance
• Revenue Vehicle Control/Dispatch
• CDL/Non-Revenue Vehicle
• Armed Security Personnel
• Ferry Boat Operator
Test Types
• Pre-employment
• Random
• Post-Accident
• Reasonable Suspicion
• Return-to-Duty
• Follow-up
Drug Types
• Marijuana
• Cocaine
• Phencyclidine (PCP)
• Opiates
• Amphetamines

1.2 Regions Required to Test

The FTA comprises 10 regions, which are identified in Figure 1. The data provided by these regions have facilitated the comparison of drug and alcohol test results and the identification of regional trends. Table 2 lists the states and territories in each FTA region.

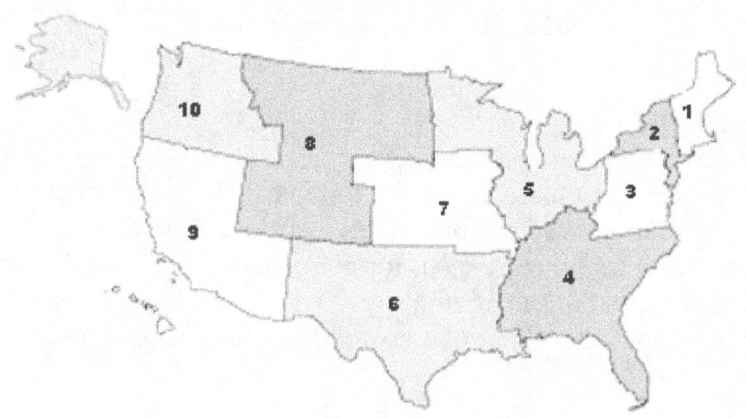

Figure 1. The Ten FTA Regions Required to Test for Drugs and Alcohol

Table 2. States and Territories by Region

Region	States
1	Connecticut, Maine, Massachusetts, New Hampshire, Rhode Island, Vermont
2	New Jersey, New York, U.S. Virgin Islands
3	Delaware, District of Columbia, Maryland, Pennsylvania, Virginia, West Virginia
4	Alabama, Florida, Georgia, Kentucky, Mississippi, North Carolina, South Carolina, Tennessee, Puerto Rico
5	Illinois, Indiana, Michigan, Minnesota, Ohio, Wisconsin
6	Arkansas, Louisiana, New Mexico, Oklahoma, Texas
7	Iowa, Kansas, Missouri, Nebraska
8	Colorado, Montana, North Dakota, South Dakota, Utah, Wyoming
9	American Samoa, Arizona, California, Guam, Hawaii, Nevada, Northern Mariana Islands
10	Alaska, Idaho, Oregon, Washington

1.3   Covered Employees and Employers

A covered employee is any person, including an applicant, transferee, or volunteer, who performs or will perform a safety-sensitive function for an entity subject to 49 Code of Federal Regulations (CFR) Part 655. A covered employer is a recipient or other entity that provides a mass transportation service or performs a safety-sensitive function for such recipient or other entity. This includes Section 5311 State Nonurban subrecipients, Section 5307 Urbanized Area Formula grantees, Section 5309 Major Capital Investment recipients, and contractors. Table 3 provides a list of the number of covered employees and employers in each FTA region.

Table 3. Number of Covered Employees and Employers by Region

Region	Number of Covered Employees	Number of Covered Employers
1	13,290	205
2	56,033	209
3	30,905	188
4	32,329	589
5	40,654	667
6	19,100	234
7	9,502	338
8	9,146	200
9	46,370	388
10	15,829	200
Total	273,158	3,218

1.4 Percent Positive for Drugs and Alcohol

When testing for drugs, the term "percent positive" refers to the number of verified positive results plus the number of refusal results divided by the number of test results. For alcohol tests, percent positive is the number of confirmation tests with results of 0.04 or greater plus the number of refusal results divided by the number of screening test results.

2. Random Drug and Alcohol Rates

2.1 Official Random Rates for 2006

Figures 2 and 3 show the official rates for random drug and alcohol tests used by the FTA Administrator in determining the random rates for 2007. Figure 2 shows the positive rate for random drug tests over the last 13 years (1995 through 2007). Figure 3 shows the violation rate for random alcohol tests over the same 13-year span.

2.2 Calculating Positive Rates and Violation Rates

The positive rate for drugs is calculated by taking the total number of verified positive tests; adding the total number of adulterated samples plus the total number of substituted specimens, shy bladder instances (those without medical explanation), and other refusals; and dividing by the total number of drug test results. The violation rate for alcohol is calculated by taking the total number of confirmatory test results greater than or equal to a breath alcohol level of 0.04, adding the total number of shy lung instances (those without medical explanation) plus the total number of other refusals, and dividing by the total number of screens conducted.

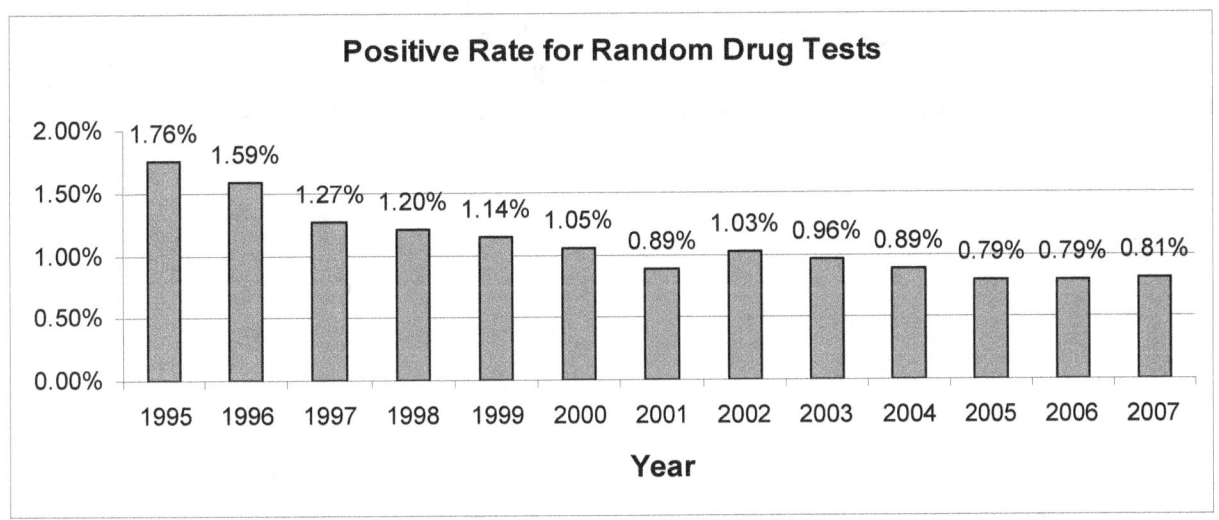

Figure 2. Positive Rate for Random Drug Tests (1995–2007)

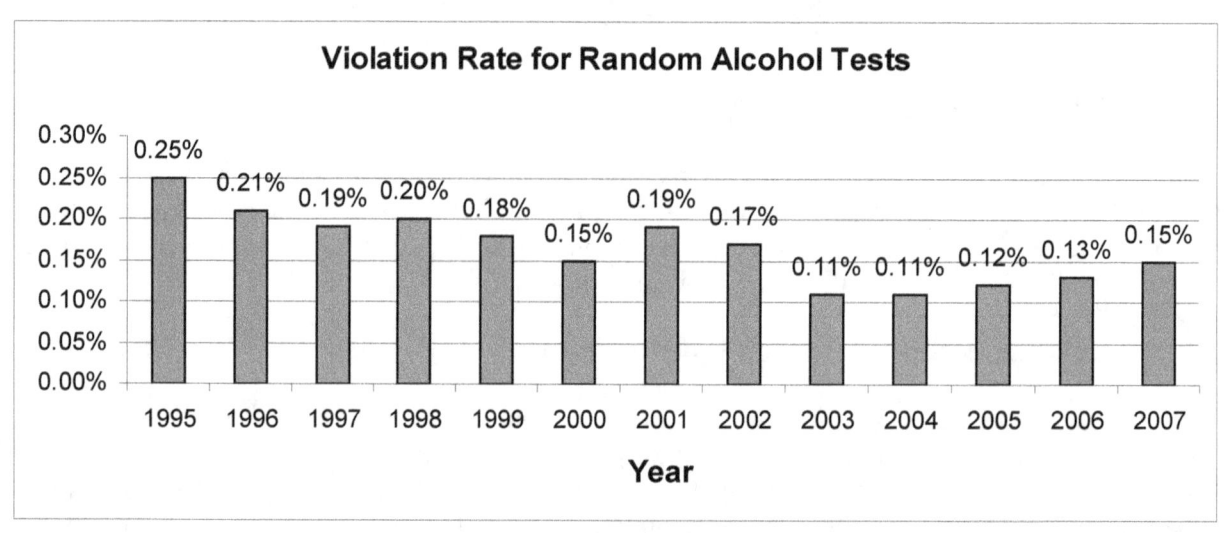

Figure 3. Violation Rate for Random Alcohol Tests (1995–2007)

2.3 Official Positive Rate and Violation Rate Trends

As shown in Figure 4, the official positive rate (drugs) increased to 0.81 percent. While the rate has increased slightly from 2006, it is still lower than the random positive rate recorded in 1995. The violation rate (alcohol) also increased slightly to 0.15 percent in 2007.

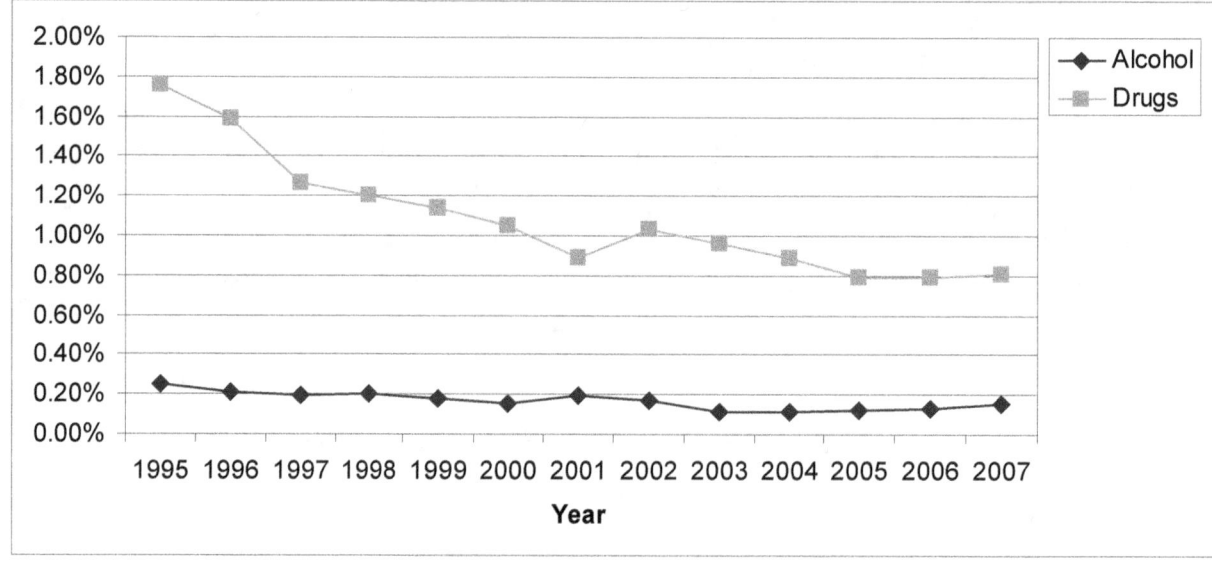

Figure 4. Official Positive Rates and Violation Rates (1995–2007)

3. Drug Test Results

3.1 Drug Test Results by Test Type

This section provides drug test results by test type conducted and for each employee category.

3.1.1 Pre-employment Drug Test Results

Table 4 provides results of pre-employment drug tests for all employee categories. Figure 5 illustrates the percent positive by employee category for all pre-employment drug tests.

Table 4. Pre-employment Drug Test Results by Employee Categories

| Employee Category | Total Number of Test Results | Verified Negative Results | Verified Positive Results for One or More Drugs | Positive for Marijuana | Positive for Cocaine | Positive for PCP | Positive for Opiates | Positive for Amphetamines | Refusals | | | | Cancelled Tests |
									Adulterated	Substituted	"Shy Bladder" with No Medical Explanation	Other Refusals to Submit to Testing	
Revenue Vehicle Operation	79,328	77,255	1,912	1,340	471	45	37	69	25	9	12	115	224
Revenue Vehicle & Equipment Maintenance	10,025	9,764	243	185	41	4	6	12	4	1	2	11	13
Revenue Vehicle Control/Dispatch	3,282	3,226	50	32	11	0	2	7	0	0	2	4	11
CDL/Non-Revenue Vehicle	879	861	17	11	3	0	1	2	1	0	0	0	0
Armed Security Personnel	1,139	1,131	6	2	4	0	0	0	0	1	0	1	2
TOTAL	94,653	92,237	2,228	1,570	530	49	46	90	30	11	16	131	250

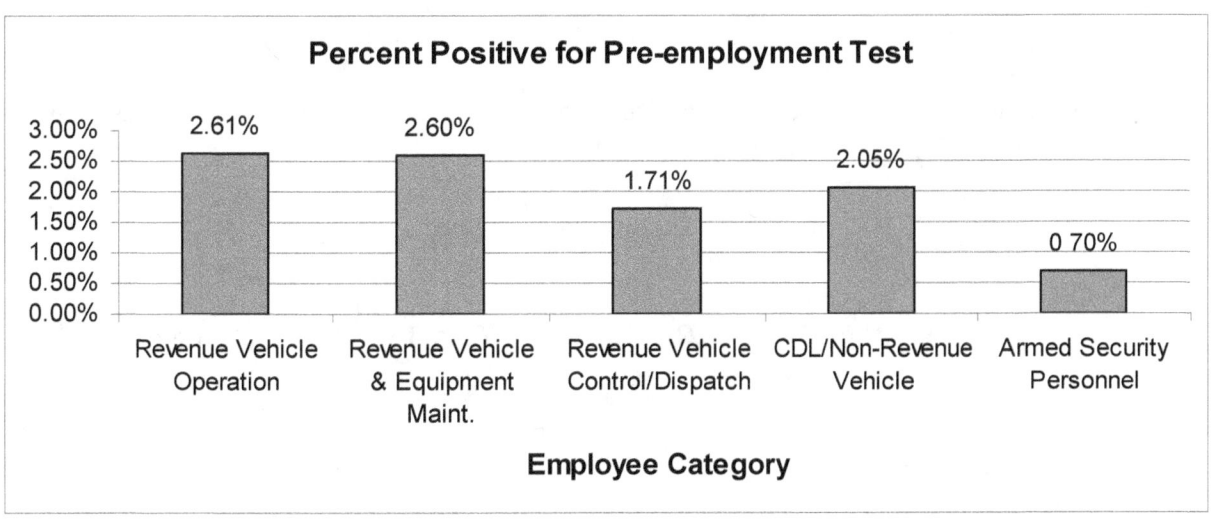

Figure 5. Percent Positive for Pre-employment Drug Tests by Employee Category

7

3.1.2 Random Drug Test Results

Table 5 provides results of random drug tests for all employee categories. Figure 6 illustrates the percent positive by employee category for all random drug tests.

Table 5. Random Drug Test Results by Employee Categories

Employee Category	Total Number of Test Results	Verified Negative Results	Verified Positive Results for One or More Drugs	Positive for Marijuana	Positive for Cocaine	Positive for PCP	Positive for Opiates	Positive for Amphetamines	Refusals				Cancelled Tests
									Adulterated	Substituted	"Shy Bladder" with No Medical Explanation	Other Refusals to Submit to Testing	
Revenue Vehicle Operation	68,405	67,832	496	278	185	8	17	25	5	4	10	58	146
Revenue Vehicle & Equipment Maintenance	17,849	17,698	140	87	52	2	2	4	0	0	3	8	23
Revenue Vehicle Control/Dispatch	6,991	6,946	41	29	9	2	0	1	0	0	0	4	13
CDL/Non-Revenue Vehicle	1,701	1,689	11	7	4	0	0	0	0	0	1	0	3
Armed Security Personnel	1,551	1,550	1	1	0	0	0	0	0	0	0	0	2
TOTAL	**96,497**	**95,715**	**689**	**402**	**250**	**12**	**19**	**30**	**5**	**4**	**14**	**70**	**187**

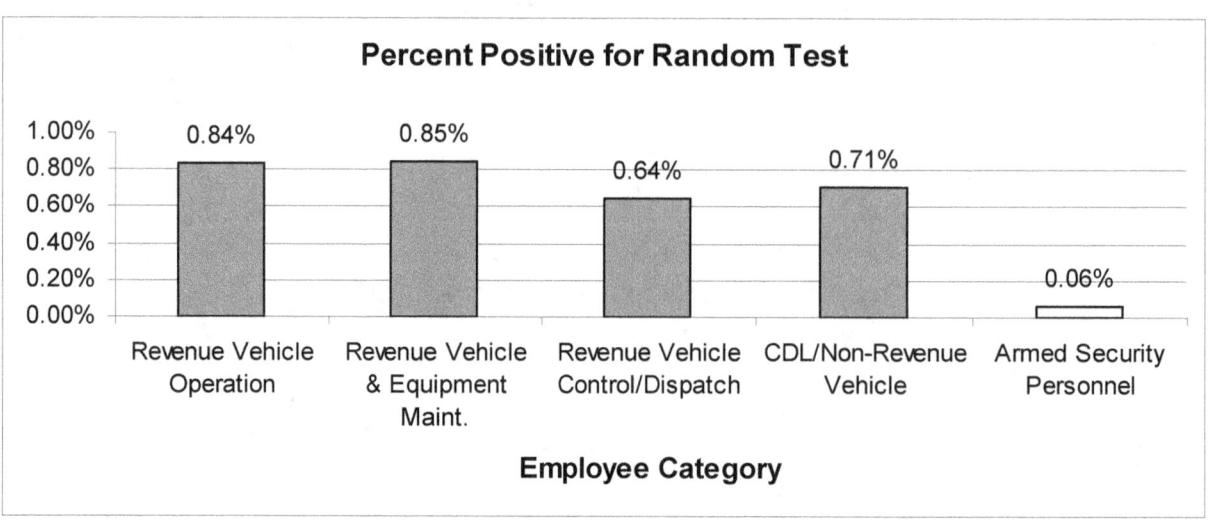

Figure 6. Percent Positive for Random Drug Tests by Employee Category

3.1.3 Post-Accident Drug Test Results

Table 6 provides results of post-accident drug tests for all employee categories. Figure 7 illustrates the percent positive by employee category for all post-accident drug tests.

Table 6. Post-Accident Drug Test Results by Employee Categories

| Employee Category | Total Number of Test Results | Verified Negative Results | Verified Positive Results for One or More Drugs | Positive for Marijuana | Positive for Cocaine | Positive for PCP | Positive for Opiates | Positive for Amphetamines | Refusals | | | | Cancelled Tests |
									Adulterated	Substituted	"Shy Bladder" with No Medical Explanation	Other Refusals to Submit to Testing	
Revenue Vehicle Operation	12,808	12,633	165	86	67	3	7	10	0	1	0	9	20
Revenue Vehicle & Equipment Maintenance	608	600	8	5	1	1	0	1	0	0	0	0	0
Revenue Vehicle Control/Dispatch	136	134	2	2	0	0	0	0	0	0	0	0	0
CDL/Non-Revenue Vehicle	76	74	1	0	1	0	0	0	0	0	0	1	0
Armed Security Personnel	83	83	0	0	0	0	0	0	0	0	0	0	0
TOTAL	13,711	13,524	176	93	69	4	7	11	0	1	0	10	20

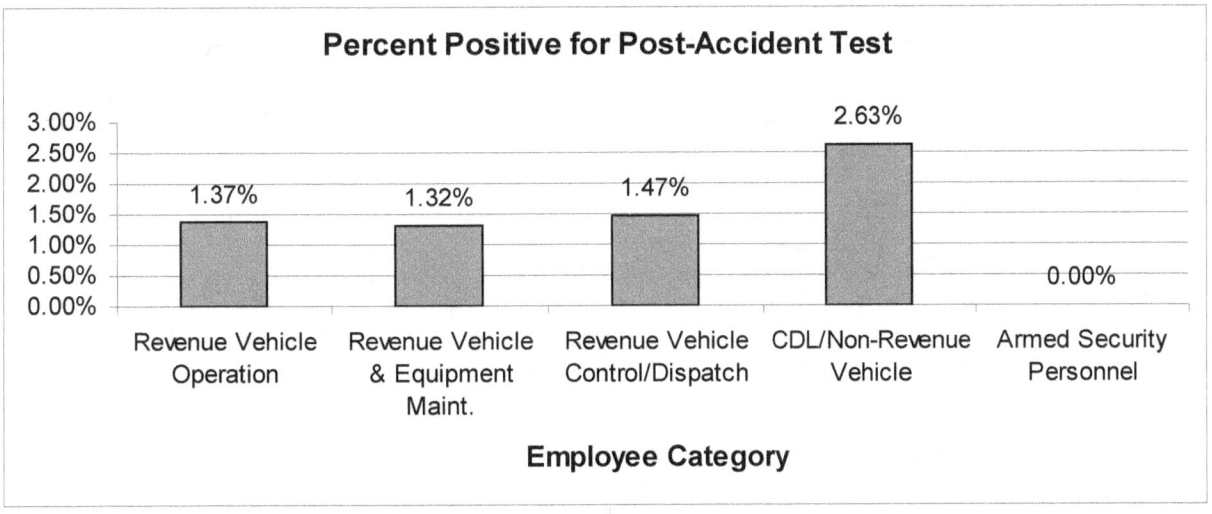

Figure 7. Percent Positive for Post-Accident Drug Tests by Employee Category

3.1.4 Reasonable Suspicion Drug Test Results

Table 7 provides results of reasonable suspicion drug tests for all employee categories. Figure 8 illustrates the percent positive by employee category for all reasonable suspicion drug tests.

Table 7. Reasonable Suspicion Drug Test Results by Employee Categories

| Employee Category | Total Number of Test Results | Verified Negative Results | Verified Positive Results for One or More Drugs | Positive for Marijuana | Positive for Cocaine | Positive for PCP | Positive for Opiates | Positive for Amphetamines | Refusals | | | | Cancelled Tests |
									Adulterated	Substituted	"Shy Bladder" with No Medical Explanation	Other Refusals to Submit to Testing	
Revenue Vehicle Operation	429	371	43	24	14	0	6	2	0	1	0	14	2
Revenue Vehicle & Equipment Maintenance	77	69	4	1	3	0	0	0	0	0	1	3	0
Revenue Vehicle Control/Dispatch	16	13	2	1	0	0	0	1	0	0	0	1	0
CDL/Non-Revenue Vehicle	5	5	0	0	0	0	0	0	0	0	0	0	2
Armed Security Personnel	3	2	0	0	0	0	0	0	0	0	0	1	0
TOTAL	530	460	49	26	17	0	6	3	0	1	1	19	4

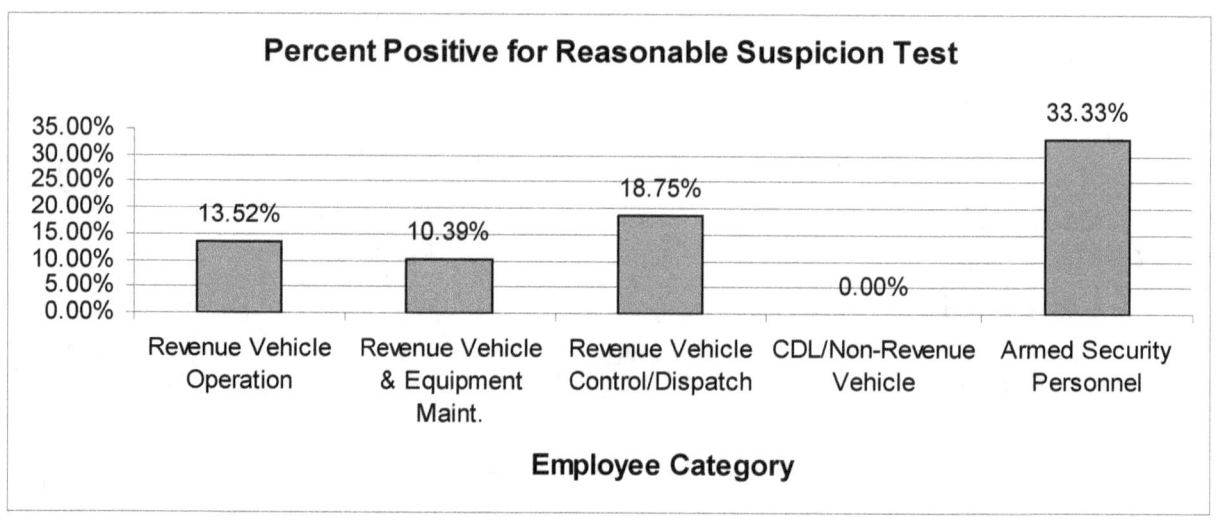

Figure 8. Percent Positive for Reasonable Suspicion Drug Tests by Employee Category

3.1.5 Return-to-Duty Drug Test Results

Table 8 provides results of return-to-duty drug tests for all employee categories. Figure 9 illustrates the percent positive by employee category for all return-to-duty drug tests.

Table 8. Return-to-Duty Drug Test Results for All Employee Categories

| Employee Category | Total Number of Test Results | Verified Negative Results | Verified Positive Results for One or More Drugs | Positive for Marijuana | Positive for Cocaine | Positive for PCP | Positive for Opiates | Positive for Amphetamines | Refusals | | | | Cancelled Tests |
									Adulterated	Substituted	"Shy Bladder" with No Medical Explanation	Other Refusals to Submit to Testing	
Revenue Vehicle Operation	716	705	11	5	5	1	1	0	0	0	0	0	1
Revenue Vehicle & Equipment Maintenance	165	163	2	1	1	0	0	0	0	0	0	0	0
Revenue Vehicle Control/Dispatch	37	37	0	0	0	0	0	0	0	0	0	0	0
CDL/Non-Revenue Vehicle	7	7	0	0	0	0	0	0	0	0	0	0	0
Armed Security Personnel	0	0	0	0	0	0	0	0	0	0	0	0	0
TOTAL	925	912	13	6	6	1	1	0	0	0	0	0	1

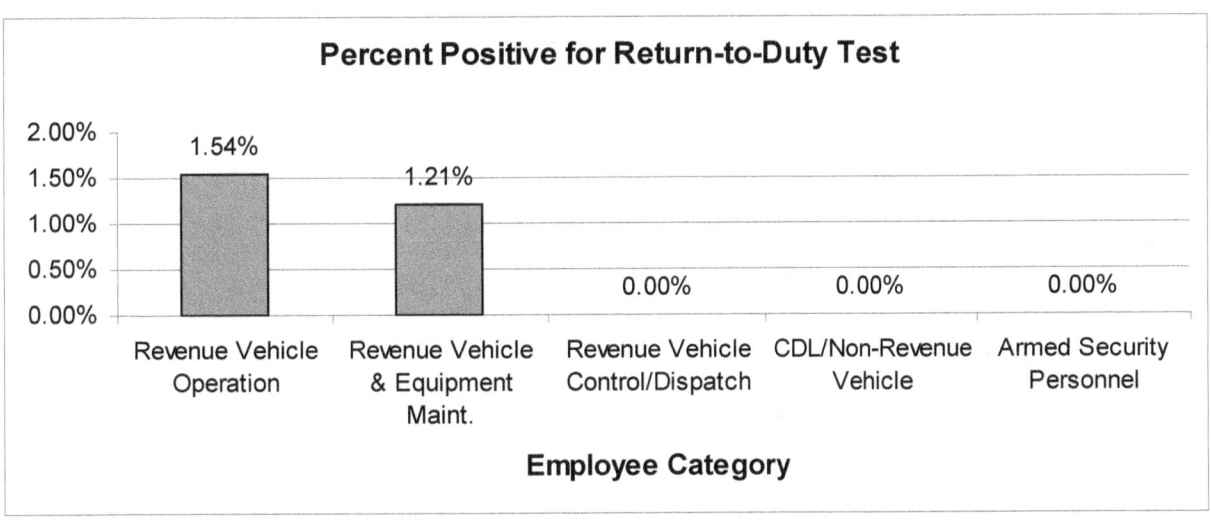

Figure 9. Percent Positive for Return-to-Duty Drug Tests by Employee Category

3.1.6 Follow-up Drug Test Results

Table 9 provides results of follow-up drug tests for all employee categories. Figure 10 illustrates the percent positive by employee category for all follow-up drug tests.

Table 9. Follow-up Drug Test Results for All Employee Categories

Employee Category	Total Number of Test Results	Verified Negative Results	Verified Positive Results for One or More Drugs	Positive for Marijuana	Positive for Cocaine	Positive for PCP	Positive for Opiates	Positive for Amphetamines	Adulterated	Substituted	"Shy Bladder" with No Medical Explanation	Other Refusals to Submit to Testing	Cancelled Tests
									Refusals				
Revenue Vehicle Operation	4,147	4,084	57	29	25	1	1	1	1	0	0	5	5
Revenue Vehicle & Equipment Maintenance	1,674	1,649	24	15	9	0	0	0	0	0	0	1	2
Revenue Vehicle Control/Dispatch	243	240	3	0	3	0	0	0	0	0	0	0	0
CDL/Non-Revenue Vehicle	145	141	4	1	0	0	3	0	0	0	0	0	0
Armed Security Personnel	23	23	0	0	0	0	0	0	0	0	0	0	0
TOTAL	**6,232**	**6,137**	**88**	**45**	**37**	**1**	**4**	**1**	**1**	**0**	**0**	**6**	**7**

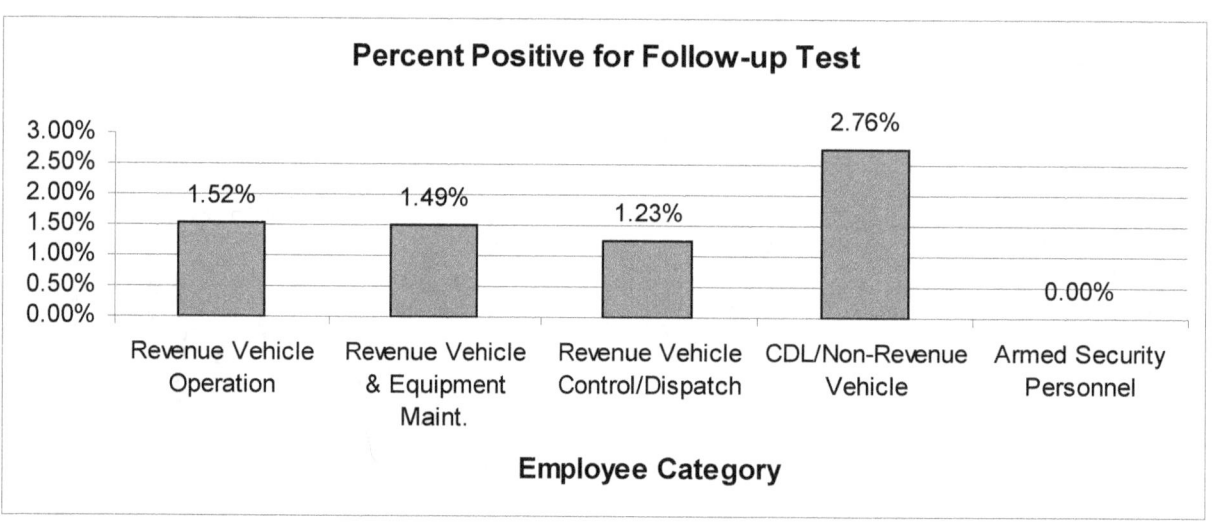

Figure 10. Percent Positive for Follow-up Drug Tests by Employee Category

12

3.1.7 Drug Test Results by Test Type for All Employee Categories

Table 10 provides drug test results by test type for all employee categories. Figure 11 illustrates the percent positive for all employee categories by test type.

Table 10. Drug Test Results by Test Type for All Employee Categories

| Test Type | Total Number of Test Results | Verified Negative Results | Verified Positive Results for One or More Drugs | Positive for Marijuana | Positive for Cocaine | Positive for PCP | Positive for Opiates | Positive for Amphetamines | Refusals | | | | Cancelled Tests |
									Adulterated	Substituted	"Shy Bladder" with No Medical Explanation	Other Refusals to Submit to Testing	
Pre-employment	94,653	92,237	2,228	1,570	530	49	46	90	30	11	16	131	250
Random	96,497	95,715	689	402	250	12	19	30	5	4	14	70	187
Post-Accident	13,711	13,524	176	93	69	4	7	11	0	1	0	10	20
Reasonable Suspicion	530	460	49	26	17	0	6	3	0	1	1	19	4
Return-to-Duty	925	912	13	6	6	1	1	0	0	0	0	0	1
Follow-up	6,232	6,137	88	45	37	1	4	1	1	0	0	6	7
TOTAL	**212,548**	**208,985**	**3,243**	**2,142**	**909**	**67**	**83**	**135**	**36**	**17**	**31**	**236**	**469**

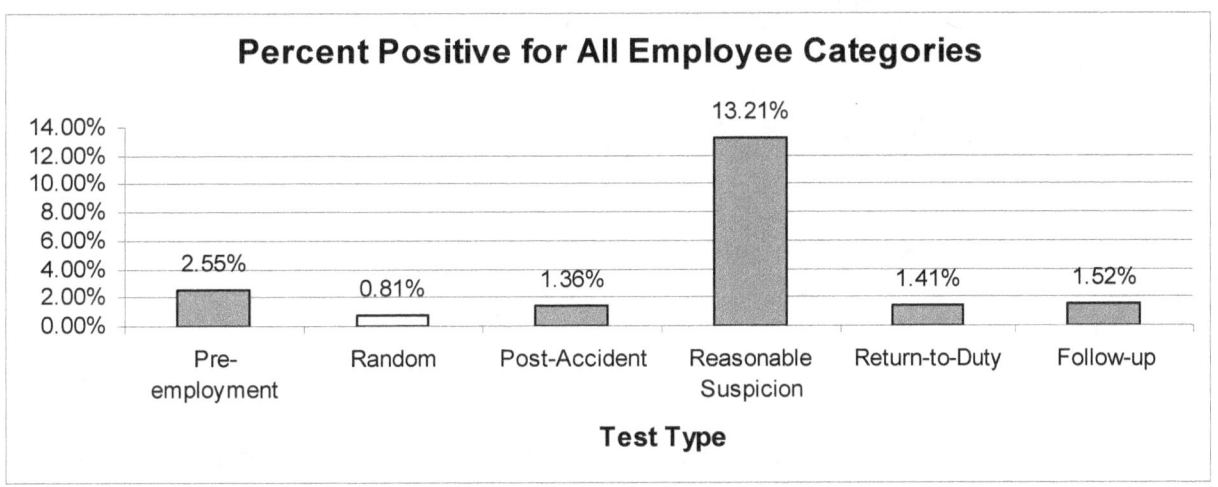

Figure 11. Percent Positive for All Employee Categories by Test Type

13

3.2 Drug Test Results by Employee Category

3.2.1 Revenue Vehicle Operation

Table 11 provides drug test results for the revenue vehicle operation employee category. Figure 12 illustrates the percent positive for each test type under the revenue vehicle operation employee category.

Table 11. Drug Test Results for Revenue Vehicle Operation

| Test Type | Total Number of Test Results | Verified Negative Results | Verified Positive Results for One or More Drugs | Positive for Marijuana | Positive for Cocaine | Positive for PCP | Positive for Opiates | Positive for Amphetamines | Refusals | | | | Cancelled Tests |
									Adulterated	Substituted	"Shy Bladder" with No Medical Explanation	Other Refusals to Submit to Testing	
Pre-employment	79,328	77,255	1,912	1,340	471	45	37	69	25	9	12	115	224
Random	68,405	67,832	496	278	185	8	17	25	5	4	10	58	146
Post-Accident	12,808	12,633	165	86	67	3	7	10	0	1	0	9	20
Reasonable Suspicion	429	371	43	24	14	0	6	2	0	1	0	14	2
Return-to-Duty	716	705	11	5	5	1	1	0	0	0	0	0	1
Follow-up	4,147	4,084	57	29	25	1	1	1	1	0	0	5	5
TOTAL	**165,833**	**162,880**	**2,684**	**1,762**	**767**	**58**	**69**	**107**	**31**	**15**	**22**	**201**	**398**

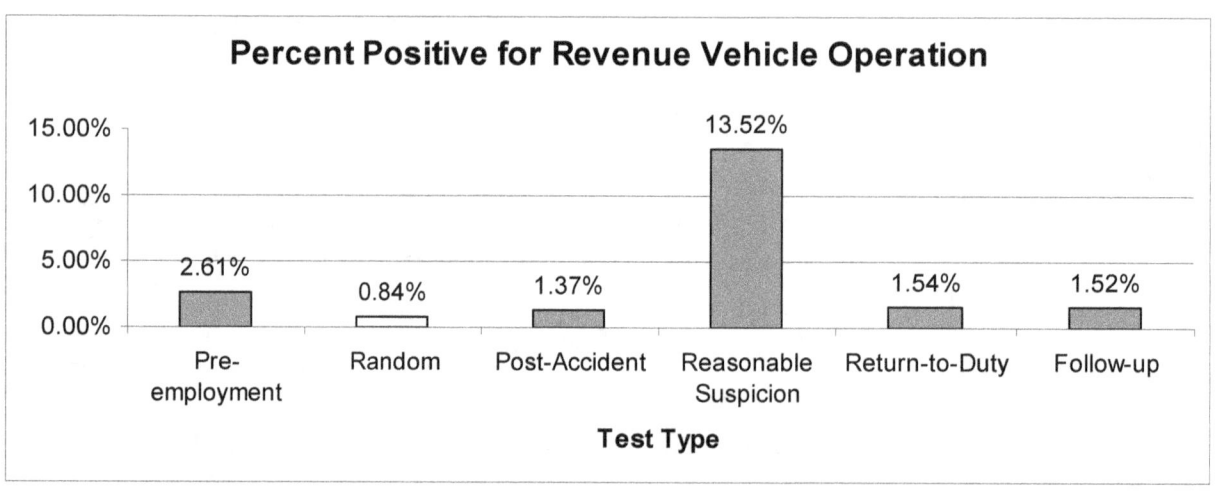

Figure 12. Percent Positive for Revenue Vehicle Operation by Test Type

14

3.2.2 Revenue Vehicle and Equipment Maintenance

Table 12 provides drug test results for the revenue vehicle and equipment maintenance employee category by test type. Figure 13 illustrates the percent positive for the revenue vehicle and equipment maintenance employee category by test type.

Table 12. Drug Test Results for Revenue Vehicle and Equipment Maintenance

| Test Type | Total Number of Test Results | Verified Negative Results | Verified Positive Results for One or More Drugs | Positive for Marijuana | Positive for Cocaine | Positive for PCP | Positive for Opiates | Positive for Amphetamines | Refusals | | | | Cancelled Tests |
									Adulterated	Substituted	"Shy Bladder" with No Medical Explanation	Other Refusals to Submit to Testing	
Pre-employment	10,025	9,764	243	185	41	4	6	12	4	1	2	11	13
Random	17,849	17,698	140	87	52	2	2	4	0	0	3	8	23
Post-Accident	608	600	8	5	1	1	0	1	0	0	0	0	0
Reasonable Suspicion	77	69	4	1	3	0	0	0	0	0	1	3	0
Return-to-Duty	165	163	2	1	1	0	0	0	0	0	0	0	0
Follow-up	1,674	1,649	24	15	9	0	0	0	0	0	0	1	2
TOTAL	**30,398**	**29,943**	**421**	**294**	**107**	**7**	**8**	**17**	**4**	**1**	**6**	**23**	**38**

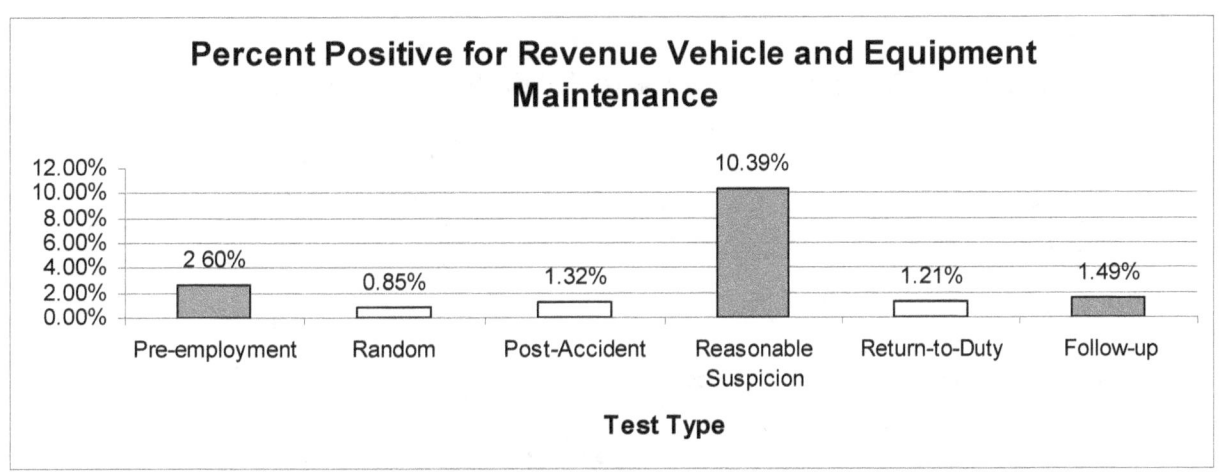

Figure 13. Percent Positive for Revenue Vehicle and Equipment Maintenance by Test Type

3.2.3 Revenue Vehicle Control/Dispatch

Table 13 provides drug test results for the revenue vehicle control/dispatch employee category by test type. Figure 14 illustrates the percent positive for the revenue vehicle control/dispatch employee category by test type.

Table 13. Drug Test Results for Revenue Vehicle Control/Dispatch

Test Type	Total Number of Test Results	Verified Negative Results	Verified Positive Results for One or More Drugs	Positive for Marijuana	Positive for Cocaine	Positive for PCP	Positive for Opiates	Positive for Amphetamines	Refusals Adulterated	Refusals Substituted	Refusals "Shy Bladder" with No Medical Explanation	Refusals Other Refusals to Submit to Testing	Cancelled Tests
Pre-employment	3,282	3,226	50	32	11	0	2	7	0	0	2	4	11
Random	6,991	6,946	41	29	9	2	0	1	0	0	0	4	13
Post-Accident	136	134	2	2	0	0	0	0	0	0	0	0	0
Reasonable Suspicion	16	13	2	1	0	0	0	1	0	0	0	1	0
Return-to-Duty	37	37	0	0	0	0	0	0	0	0	0	0	0
Follow-up	243	240	3	0	3	0	0	0	0	0	0	0	0
TOTAL	**10,705**	**10,596**	**98**	**64**	**23**	**2**	**2**	**9**	**0**	**0**	**2**	**9**	**24**

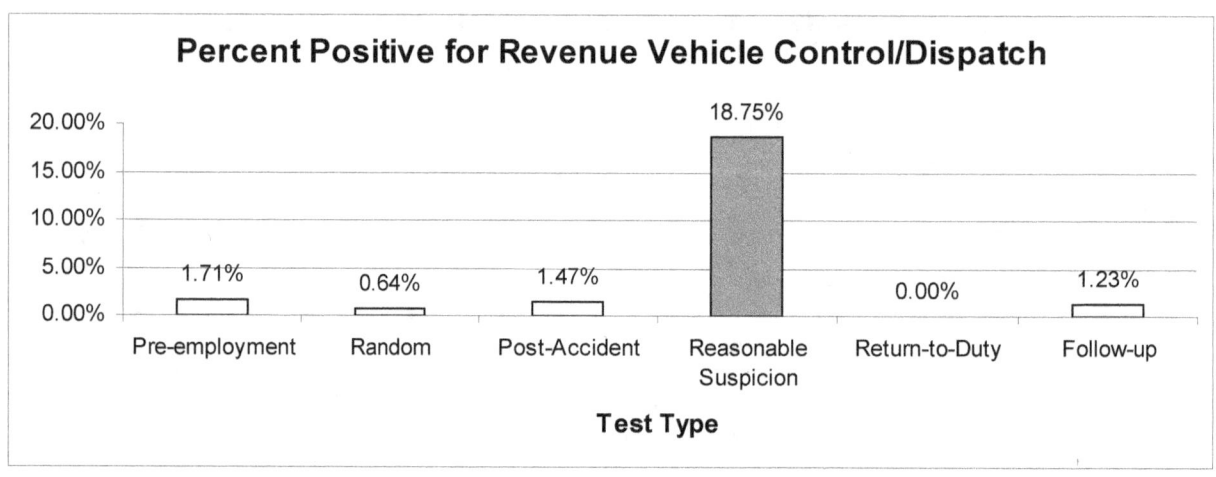

Figure 14. Percent Positive for Revenue Vehicle Control/Dispatch by Test Type

3.2.4 Commercial Driver's License (CDL)/Non-Revenue Vehicle

Table 14 provides drug test results for the commercial driver's license (CDL)/non-revenue vehicle employee category by test type. Figure 15 illustrates the percent positive for the CDL/non-revenue vehicle employee category by test type.

Table 14. Drug Test Results for Commercial Driver's License (CDL)/Non-Revenue Vehicle

| Test Type | Total Number of Test Results | Verified Negative Results | Verified Positive Results for One or More Drugs | Positive for Marijuana | Positive for Cocaine | Positive for PCP | Positive for Opiates | Positive for Amphetamines | Refusals | | | | Cancelled Tests |
									Adulterated	Substituted	"Shy Bladder" with No Medical Explanation	Other Refusals to Submit to Testing	
Pre-employment	879	861	17	11	3	0	1	2	1	0	0	0	0
Random	1,701	1,689	11	7	4	0	0	0	0	0	1	0	3
Post-Accident	76	74	1	0	1	0	0	0	0	0	0	1	0
Reasonable Suspicion	5	5	0	0	0	0	0	0	0	0	0	0	2
Return-to-Duty	7	7	0	0	0	0	0	0	0	0	0	0	0
Follow-up	145	141	4	1	0	0	3	0	0	0	0	0	0
TOTAL	**2,813**	**2,777**	**33**	**19**	**8**	**0**	**4**	**2**	**1**	**0**	**1**	**1**	**5**

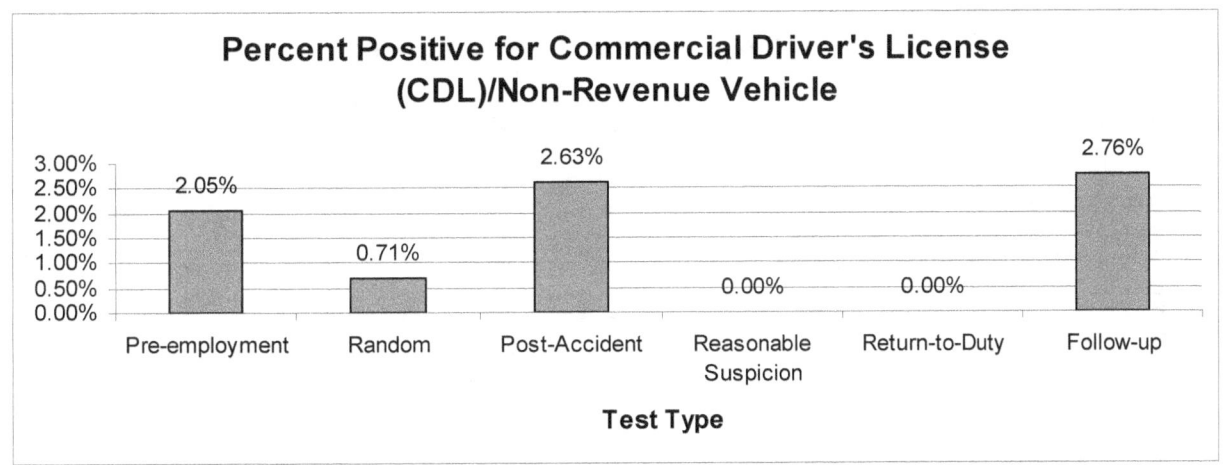

Figure 15. Percent Positive for Commercial Driver's License (CDL)/ Non-Revenue Vehicle by Test Type

3.2.5 Armed Security Personnel

Table 15 provides drug test results for the armed security personnel employee category by test type. Figure 16 illustrates the percent positive for the armed security personnel employee category by test type.

Table 15. Drug Test Results for Armed Security Personnel

Test Type	Total Number of Test Results	Verified Negative Results	Verified Positive Results for One or More Drugs	Positive for Marijuana	Positive for Cocaine	Positive for PCP	Positive for Opiates	Positive for Amphetamines	Refusals				Cancelled Tests
									Adulterated	Substituted	"Shy Bladder" with No Medical Explanation	Other Refusals to Submit to Testing	
Pre-employment	1,139	1,131	6	2	4	0	0	0	0	1	0	1	2
Random	1,551	1,550	1	1	0	0	0	0	0	0	0	0	2
Post-Accident	83	83	0	0	0	0	0	0	0	0	0	0	0
Reasonable Suspicion	3	2	0	0	0	0	0	0	0	0	0	1	0
Return-to-Duty	0	0	0	0	0	0	0	0	0	0	0	0	0
Follow-up	23	23	0	0	0	0	0	0	0	0	0	0	0
TOTAL	**2,799**	**2,789**	**7**	**3**	**4**	**0**	**0**	**0**	**0**	**1**	**0**	**2**	**4**

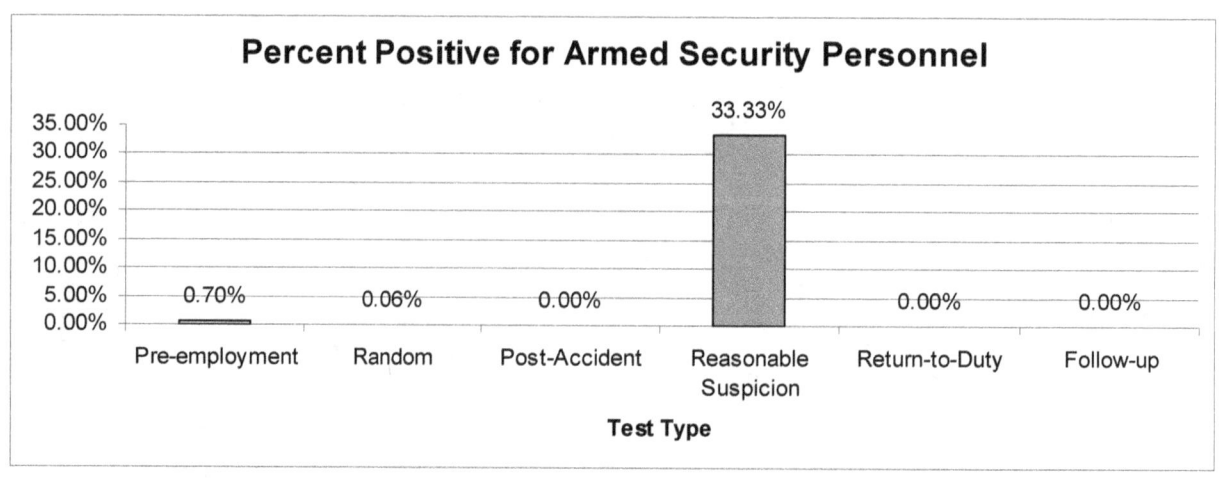

Figure 16. Percent Positive for Armed Security Personnel by Test Type

3.2.6 Drug Test Results for All Employee Categories

Table 16 provides drug test results for all test types by employee category. Figure 17 illustrates the percent positive for all test types by employee category.

Table 16. Drug Test Results for All Test Types by Employee Category

Employee Category	Total Number of Test Results	Verified Negative Results	Verified Positive Results for One or More Drugs	Positive for Marijuana	Positive for Cocaine	Positive for PCP	Positive for Opiates	Positive for Amphetamines	Refusals				Cancelled Tests
									Adulterated	Substituted	"Shy Bladder" with No Medical Explanation	Other Refusals to Submit to Testing	
Revenue Vehicle Operation	165,833	162,880	2,684	1,762	767	58	69	107	31	15	22	201	398
Revenue Vehicle & Equipment Maintenance	30,398	29,943	421	294	107	7	8	17	4	1	6	23	38
Revenue Vehicle Control/Dispatch	10,705	10,596	98	64	23	2	2	9	0	0	2	9	24
CDL/Non-Revenue Vehicle	2,813	2,777	33	19	8	0	4	2	1	0	1	1	5
Armed Security Personnel	2,799	2,789	7	3	4	0	0	0	0	1	0	2	4
TOTAL	212,548	208,985	3,243	2,142	909	67	83	135	36	17	31	236	469

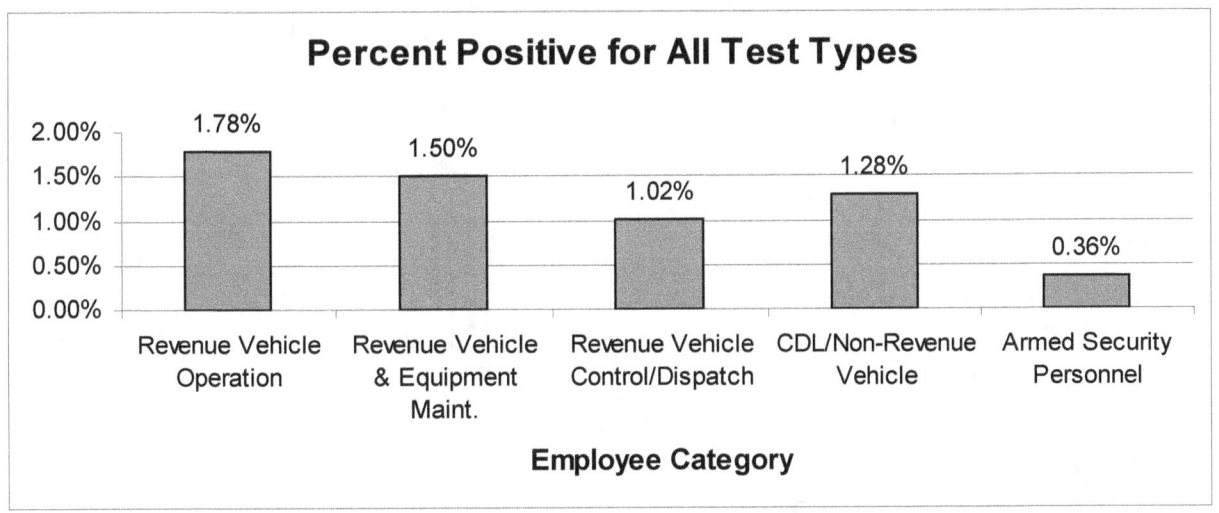

Figure 17. Percent Positive for All Test Types by Employee Category

19

3.3 Drug Test Results by Region

3.3.1 Drug Test Results for Region 1

Table 17 provides drug test results by test type and drugs detected for Region 1. Figure 18 illustrates the percent positive for all test types for Region 1.

Table 17. Drug Test Results by Test Type and Drugs Detected for Region 1

| Test Type | Total Number of Test Results | Verified Negative Results | Verified Positive Results for One or More Drugs | Positive for Marijuana | Positive for Cocaine | Positive for PCP | Positive for Opiates | Positive for Amphetamines | Refusals | | | | Cancelled Tests |
									Adulterated	Substituted	"Shy Bladder" with No Medical Explanation	Other Refusals to Submit to Testing	
Pre-employment	3,407	3,316	88	65	23	1	1	1	0	0	0	3	3
Random	4,237	4,204	30	16	14	0	0	1	0	0	0	3	22
Post-Accident	490	483	7	4	3	0	0	0	0	0	0	0	1
Reasonable Suspicion	18	12	5	4	1	0	0	0	0	0	0	1	0
Return-to-Duty	51	50	1	1	0	0	0	0	0	0	0	0	0
Follow-up	354	348	6	2	4	0	0	0	0	0	0	0	0
TOTAL	**8,557**	**8,413**	**137**	**92**	**45**	**1**	**1**	**2**	**0**	**0**	**0**	**7**	**26**

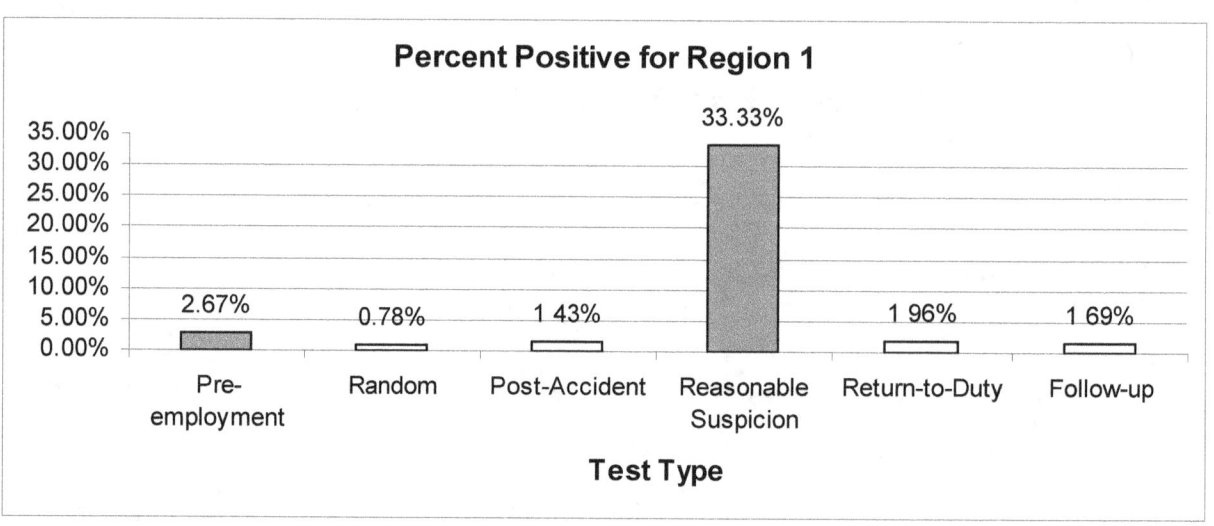

Figure 18. Percent Positive for All Test Types for Region 1

3.3.2 Drug Test Results for Region 2

Table 18 provides drug test results by test type and drugs detected for Region 2. Figure 19 illustrates the percent positive for all test types for Region 2.

Table 18. Drug Test Results by Test Type and Drugs Detected for Region 2

Test Type	Total Number of Test Results	Verified Negative Results	Verified Positive Results for One or More Drugs	Positive for Marijuana	Positive for Cocaine	Positive for PCP	Positive for Opiates	Positive for Amphetamines	Adulterated	Substituted	"Shy Bladder" with No Medical Explanation	Other Refusals to Submit to Testing	Cancelled Tests
									| Refusals |				
Pre-employment	16,311	15,917	384	271	105	7	10	2	6	2	0	2	18
Random	17,784	17,675	100	54	43	0	2	1	1	0	0	8	21
Post-Accident	2,433	2,407	24	8	16	0	0	0	0	0	0	2	2
Reasonable Suspicion	62	50	8	1	6	0	1	0	0	0	0	4	1
Return-to-Duty	156	155	1	0	1	0	0	0	0	0	0	0	0
Follow-up	1,758	1,744	14	9	5	0	0	0	0	0	0	0	1
TOTAL	**38,504**	**37,948**	**531**	**343**	**176**	**7**	**13**	**3**	**7**	**2**	**0**	**16**	**43**

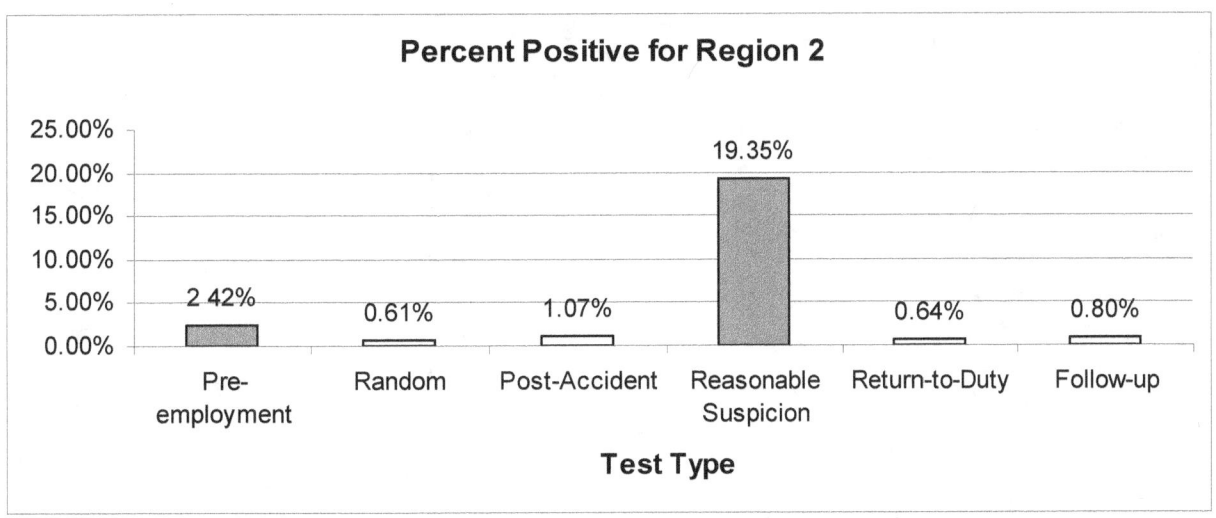

Figure 19 data:
- Pre-employment: 2.42%
- Random: 0.61%
- Post-Accident: 1.07%
- Reasonable Suspicion: 19.35%
- Return-to-Duty: 0.64%
- Follow-up: 0.80%

Figure 19. Percent Positive for All Test Types for Region 2

3.3.3 Drug Test Results for Region 3

Table 19 provides drug test results by test type and drugs detected for Region 3. Figure 20 illustrates the percent positive for all test types for Region 3.

Table 19. Drug Test Results by Test Type and Drugs Detected for Region 3

| Test Type | Total Number of Test Results | Verified Negative Results | Verified Positive Results for One or More Drugs | Positive for Marijuana | Positive for Cocaine | Positive for PCP | Positive for Opiates | Positive for Amphetamines | Refusals | | | | Cancelled Tests |
									Adulterated	Substituted	"Shy Bladder" with No Medical Explanation	Other Refusals to Submit to Testing	
Pre-employment	11,316	10,836	426	304	95	33	4	3	1	0	4	49	45
Random	11,645	11,528	106	57	37	8	6	1	1	0	0	10	18
Post-Accident	1,187	1,171	16	5	9	1	1	0	0	0	0	0	2
Reasonable Suspicion	97	84	11	5	4	0	4	0	0	0	0	2	0
Return-to-Duty	159	159	0	0	0	0	0	0	0	0	0	0	0
Follow-up	1,114	1,103	11	5	6	0	0	0	0	0	0	0	0
TOTAL	**25,518**	**24,881**	**570**	**376**	**151**	**42**	**15**	**4**	**2**	**0**	**4**	**61**	**65**

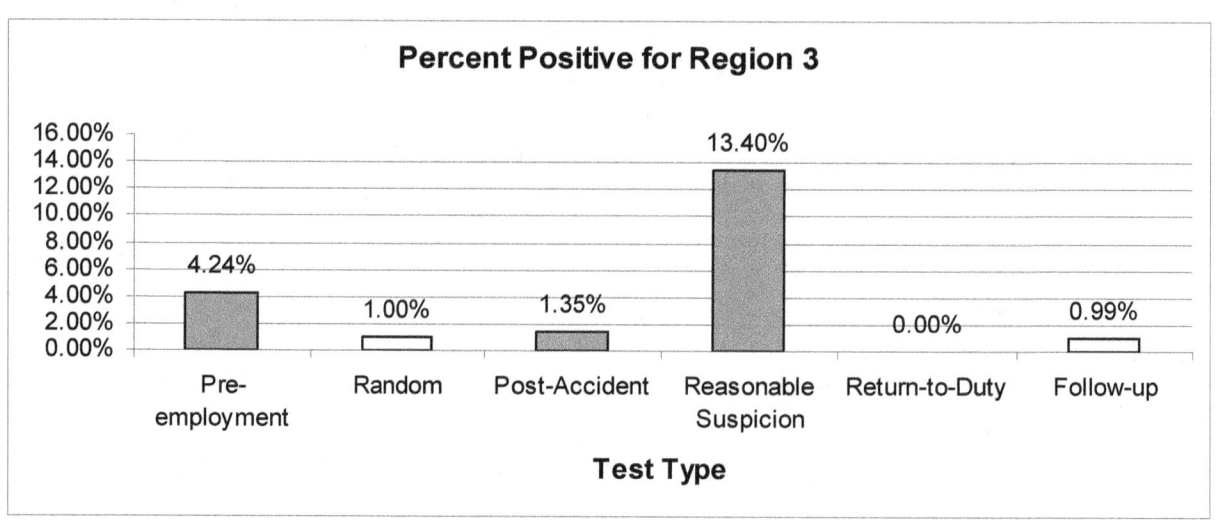

Figure 20. Percent Positive for All Test Types for Region 3

3.3.4 Drug Test Results for Region 4

Table 20 provides drug test results by test type and drugs detected for Region 4. Figure 21 illustrates the percent positive for all test types for Region 4.

Table 20. Drug Test Results by Test Type and Drugs Detected for Region 4

| Test Type | Total Number of Test Results | Verified Negative Results | Verified Positive Results for One or More Drugs | Positive for Marijuana | Positive for Cocaine | Positive for PCP | Positive for Opiates | Positive for Amphetamines | Refusals | | | | Cancelled Tests |
									Adulterated	Substituted	"Shy Bladder" with No Medical Explanation	Other Refusals to Submit to Testing	
Pre-employment	11,559	11,285	252	169	81	2	8	1	5	3	3	11	32
Random	13,224	13,117	95	62	33	1	5	2	1	0	3	8	39
Post-Accident	2,060	2,028	28	18	9	1	3	1	0	1	0	3	5
Reasonable Suspicion	59	51	5	2	3	0	0	1	0	0	0	3	2
Return-to-Duty	134	133	1	1	0	0	0	0	0	0	0	0	0
Follow-up	333	316	16	8	8	0	0	0	0	0	0	1	0
TOTAL	27,369	26,930	397	260	134	4	16	5	6	4	6	26	78

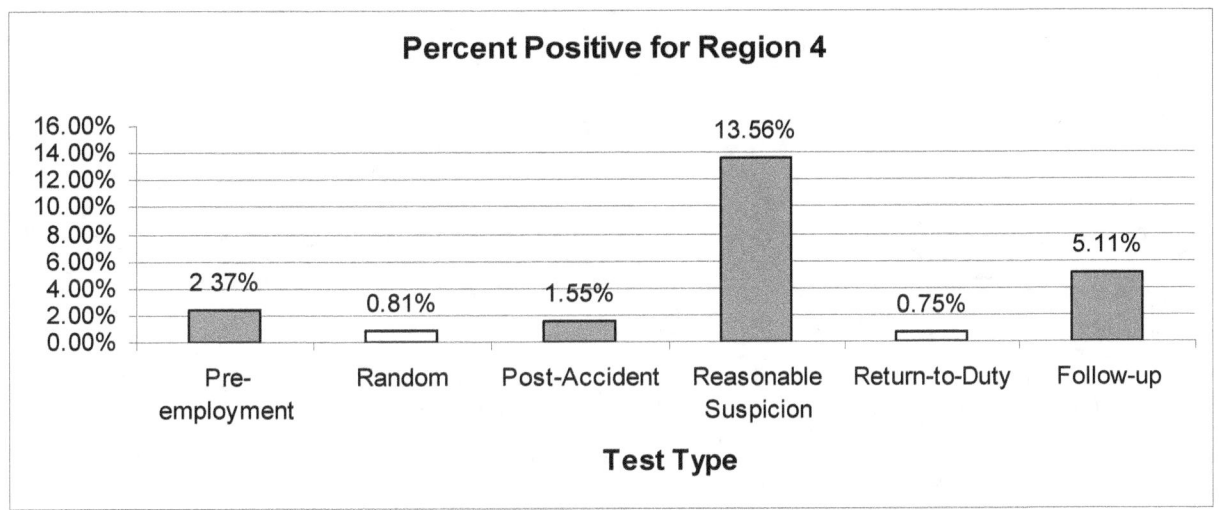

Figure 21. Percent Positive for All Test Types for Region 4

3.3.5 Drug Test Results for Region 5

Table 21 provides drug test results by test type and drugs detected for Region 5. Figure 22 illustrates the percent positive for all test types for Region 5.

Table 21. Drug Test Results by Test Type and Drugs Detected for Region 5

Test Type	Total Number of Test Results	Verified Negative Results	Verified Positive Results for One or More Drugs	Positive for Marijuana	Positive for Cocaine	Positive for PCP	Positive for Opiates	Positive for Amphetamines	Refusals				Cancelled Tests
									Adulterated	Substituted	"Shy Bladder" with No Medical Explanation	Other Refusals to Submit to Testing	
Pre-employment	11,834	11,558	254	187	64	0	5	2	9	3	2	8	19
Random	13,962	13,839	107	59	46	1	2	1	0	1	7	8	24
Post-Accident	2,532	2,488	43	21	18	1	3	0	0	0	0	1	1
Reasonable Suspicion	123	114	2	1	1	0	0	0	0	1	1	5	0
Return-to-Duty	143	139	4	2	3	0	0	0	0	0	0	0	0
Follow-up	850	840	9	4	3	0	2	0	0	0	0	1	1
TOTAL	**29,444**	**28,978**	**419**	**274**	**135**	**2**	**12**	**3**	**9**	**5**	**10**	**23**	**45**

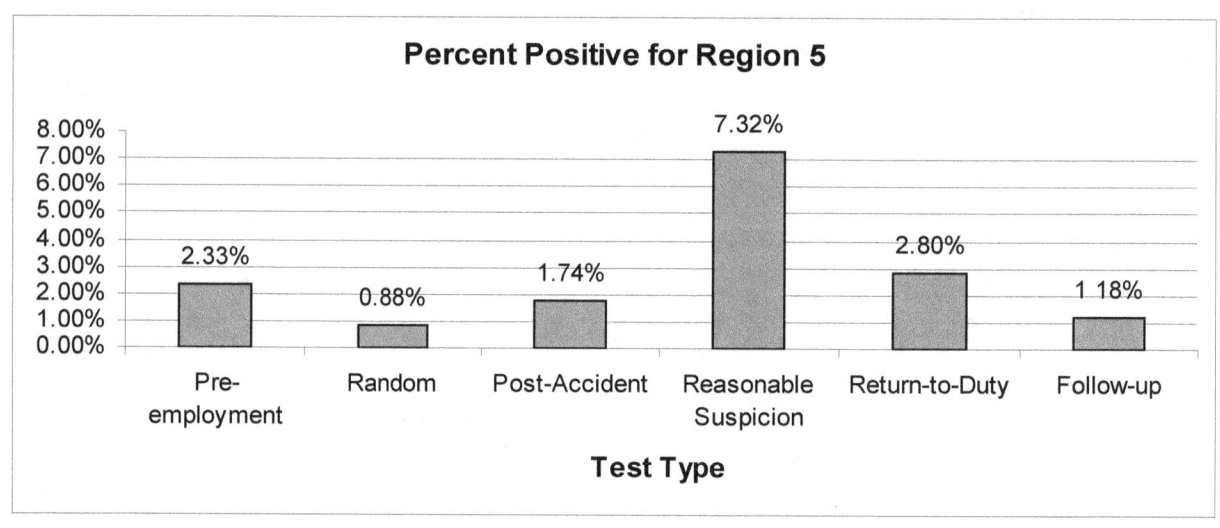

Figure 22. Percent Positive for All Test Types for Region 5

3.3.6　Drug Test Results for Region 6

Table 22 provides drug test results by test type and drugs detected for Region 6. Figure 23 illustrates the percent positive for all test types for Region 6.

Table 22. Drug Test Results by Test Type and Drugs Detected for Region 6

Test Type	Total Number of Test Results	Verified Negative Results	Verified Positive Results for One or More Drugs	Positive for Marijuana	Positive for Cocaine	Positive for PCP	Positive for Opiates	Positive for Amphetamines	Refusals				Cancelled Tests
									Adulterated	Substituted	"Shy Bladder" with No Medical Explanation	Other Refusals to Submit to Testing	
Pre-employment	7,549	7,364	159	105	49	1	0	6	2	0	3	21	20
Random	7,296	7,227	55	27	25	2	0	2	0	0	0	14	13
Post-Accident	1,034	1,019	13	8	3	1	0	1	0	0	0	2	1
Reasonable Suspicion	23	21	2	0	0	0	0	2	0	0	0	0	1
Return-to-Duty	24	21	3	2	0	1	0	0	0	0	0	0	0
Follow-up	137	132	5	1	3	1	0	0	0	0	0	0	0
TOTAL	**16,063**	**15,784**	**237**	**143**	**80**	**6**	**0**	**11**	**2**	**0**	**3**	**37**	**35**

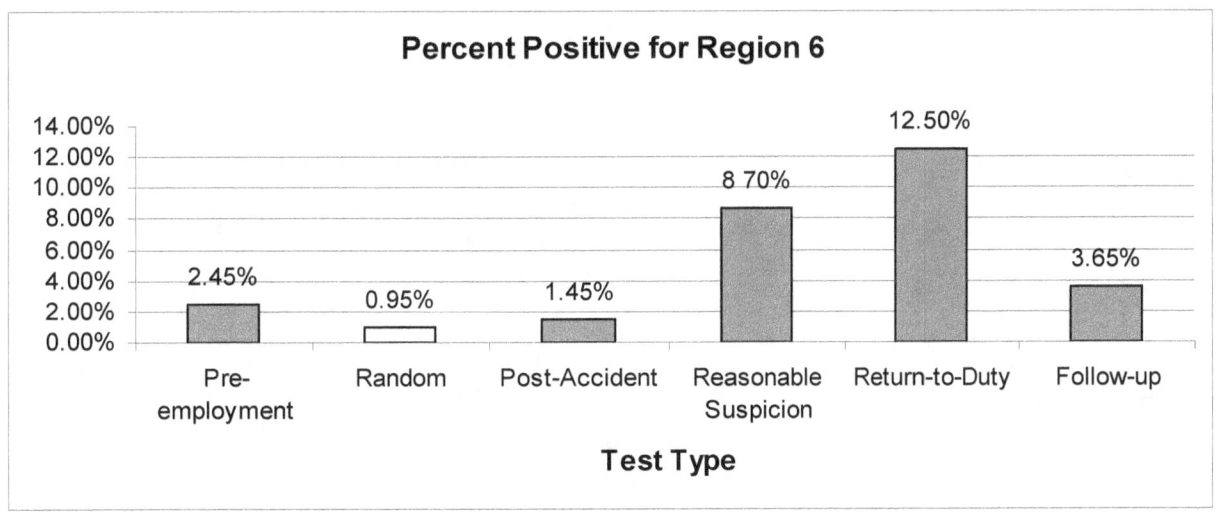

Figure 23. Percent Positive for All Test Types for Region 6

3.3.7 Drug Test Results for Region 7

Table 23 provides drug test results by test type and drugs detected for Region 7. Figure 24 illustrates the percent positive for all test types for Region 7.

Table 23. Drug Test Results by Test Type and Drugs Detected for Region 7

Test Type	Total Number of Test Results	Verified Negative Results	Verified Positive Results for One or More Drugs	Positive for Marijuana	Positive for Cocaine	Positive for PCP	Positive for Opiates	Positive for Amphetamines	Refusals Adulterated	Substituted	"Shy Bladder" with No Medical Explanation	Other Refusals to Submit to Testing	Cancelled Tests
Pre-employment	3,221	3,170	48	37	5	0	2	4	0	0	0	3	8
Random	3,491	3,464	22	17	6	0	0	0	0	0	0	5	11
Post-Accident	435	433	2	2	0	0	0	0	0	0	0	0	0
Reasonable Suspicion	17	14	2	2	0	0	0	0	0	0	0	1	0
Return-to-Duty	35	34	1	0	1	0	0	0	0	0	0	0	0
Follow-up	71	68	3	3	0	0	0	0	0	0	0	0	0
TOTAL	**7,270**	**7,183**	**78**	**61**	**12**	**0**	**2**	**4**	**0**	**0**	**0**	**9**	**19**

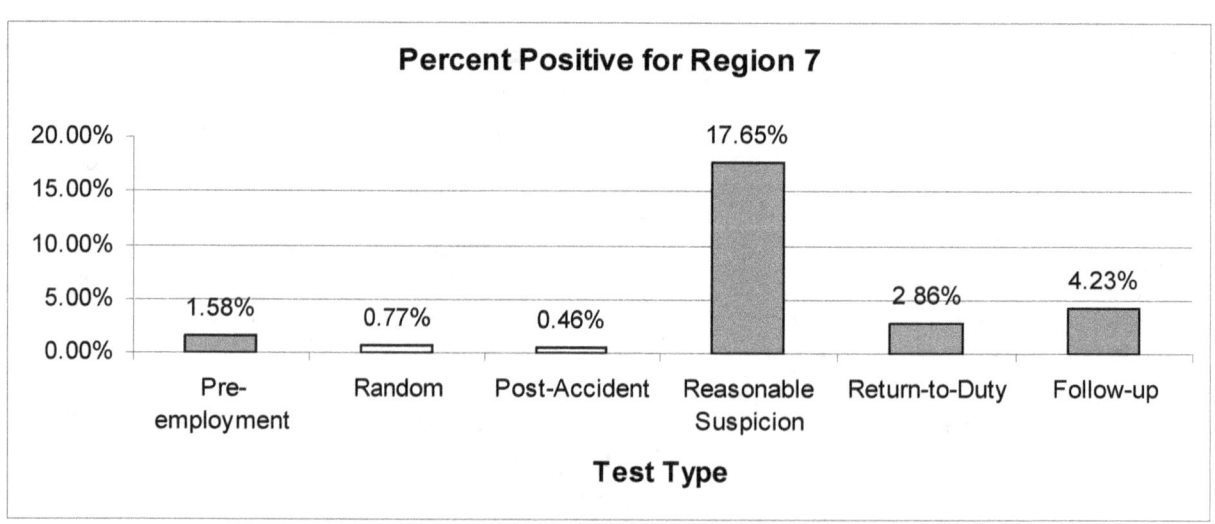

Figure 24. Percent Positive for All Test Types for Region 7

3.3.8 Drug Test Results for Region 8

Table 24 provides drug test results by test type and drugs detected for Region 8. Figure 25 illustrates the percent positive for all test types for Region 8.

Table 24. Drug Test Results by Test Type and Drugs Detected for Region 8

Test Type	Total Number of Test Results	Verified Negative Results	Verified Positive Results for One or More Drugs	Positive for Marijuana	Positive for Cocaine	Positive for PCP	Positive for Opiates	Positive for Amphetamines	Refusals				Cancelled Tests
									Adulterated	Substituted	"Shy Bladder" with No Medical Explanation	Other Refusals to Submit to Testing	
Pre-employment	4,593	4,496	94	62	27	0	3	5	1	0	0	2	13
Random	3,378	3,342	31	21	8	0	1	3	1	1	0	3	10
Post-Accident	317	313	3	2	1	0	0	0	0	0	0	1	1
Reasonable Suspicion	21	19	1	1	0	0	0	0	0	0	0	1	0
Return-to-Duty	40	39	1	0	1	0	0	0	0	0	0	0	1
Follow-up	92	91	1	1	0	0	0	0	0	0	0	0	1
TOTAL	**8,441**	**8,300**	**131**	**87**	**37**	**0**	**4**	**8**	**2**	**1**	**0**	**7**	**26**

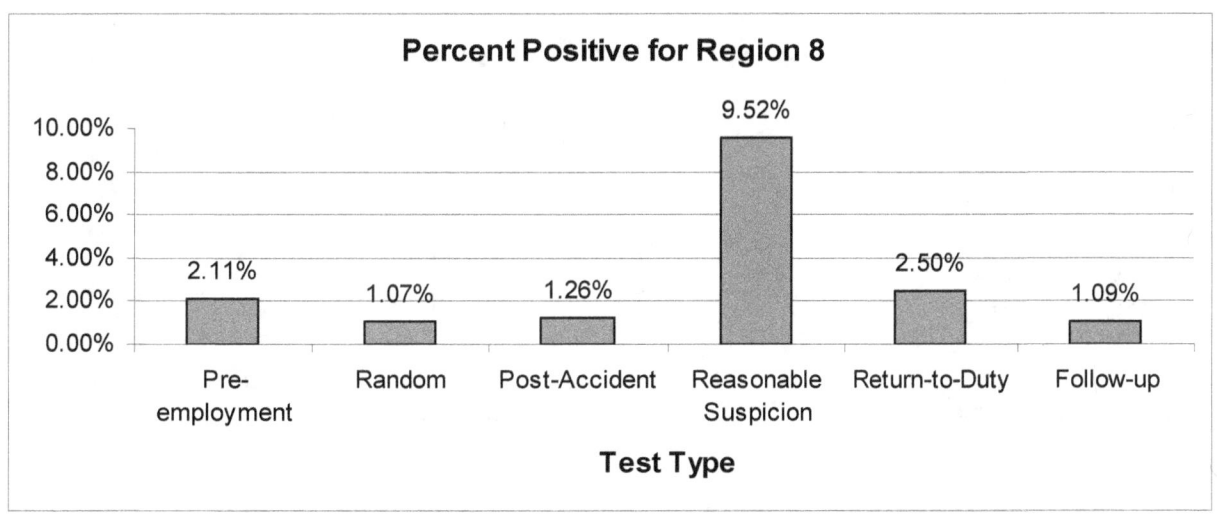

Figure 25. Percent Positive for All Test Types for Region 8

3.3.9 Drug Test Results for Region 9

Table 25 provides drug test results by test type and drugs detected for Region 9. Figure 26 illustrates the percent positive for all test types for Region 9.

Table 25. Drug Test Results by Test Type and Drugs Detected for Region 9

Test Type	Total Number of Test Results	Verified Negative Results	Verified Positive Results for One or More Drugs	Positive for Marijuana	Positive for Cocaine	Positive for PCP	Positive for Opiates	Positive for Amphetamines	Refusals				Cancelled Tests
									Adulterated	Substituted	"Shy Bladder" with No Medical Explanation	Other Refusals to Submit to Testing	
Pre-employment	20,869	20,350	481	346	74	5	13	55	6	3	4	25	91
Random	16,838	16,707	117	69	33	0	2	17	1	1	2	10	25
Post-Accident	2,625	2,588	36	22	9	0	0	9	0	0	0	1	6
Reasonable Suspicion	87	76	9	9	0	0	0	0	0	0	0	2	0
Return-to-Duty	157	156	1	0	0	0	1	0	0	0	0	0	0
Follow-up	1,285	1,261	20	11	7	0	2	0	1	0	0	3	4
TOTAL	**41,861**	**41,138**	**664**	**457**	**123**	**5**	**18**	**81**	**8**	**4**	**6**	**41**	**126**

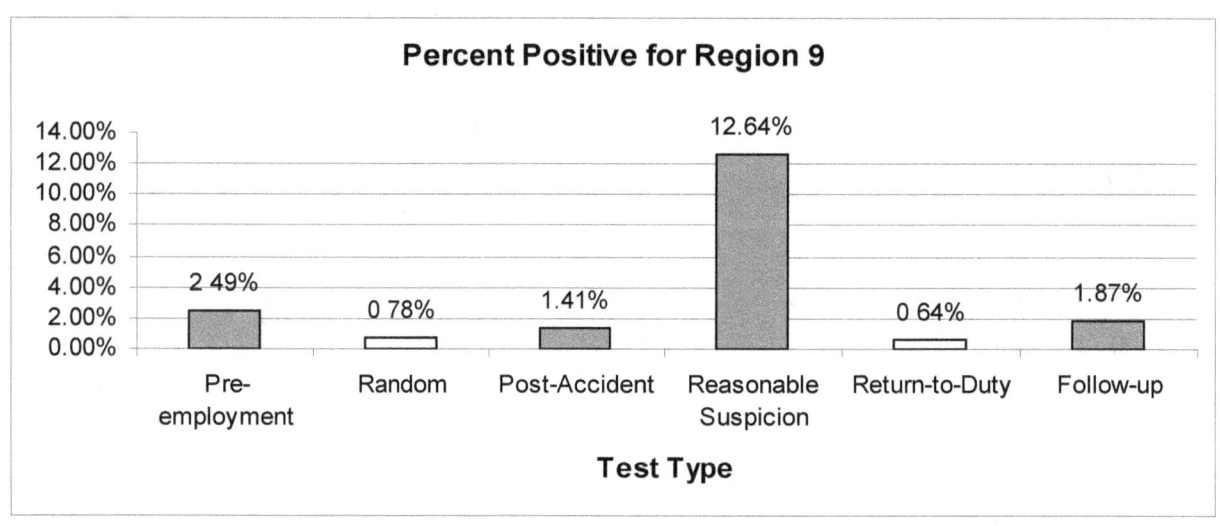

Figure 26. Percent Positive for All Test Types for Region 9

3.3.10 Drug Test Results for Region 10

Table 26 provides drug test results by test type and drugs detected for Region 10. Figure 27 illustrates the percent positive for all test types for Region 10.

Table 26. Drug Test Results by Test Type and Drugs Detected for Region 10

Test Type	Total Number of Test Results	Verified Negative Results	Verified Positive Results for One or More Drugs	Positive for Marijuana	Positive for Cocaine	Positive for PCP	Positive for Opiates	Positive for Amphetamines	Refusals Adulterated	Refusals Substituted	Refusals "Shy Bladder" with No Medical Explanation	Refusals Other Refusals to Submit to Testing	Cancelled Tests
Pre-employment	3,908	3,860	41	23	7	0	0	11	0	0	0	7	3
Random	4,588	4,558	26	20	5	0	1	2	0	1	2	1	9
Post-Accident	598	594	4	3	1	0	0	0	0	0	0	0	1
Reasonable Suspicion	22	18	4	1	2	0	1	0	0	0	0	0	0
Return-to-Duty	25	25	0	0	0	0	0	0	0	0	0	0	0
Follow-up	238	234	3	1	1	0	0	1	0	0	0	1	0
TOTAL	**9,379**	**9,289**	**78**	**48**	**16**	**0**	**2**	**14**	**0**	**1**	**2**	**9**	**13**

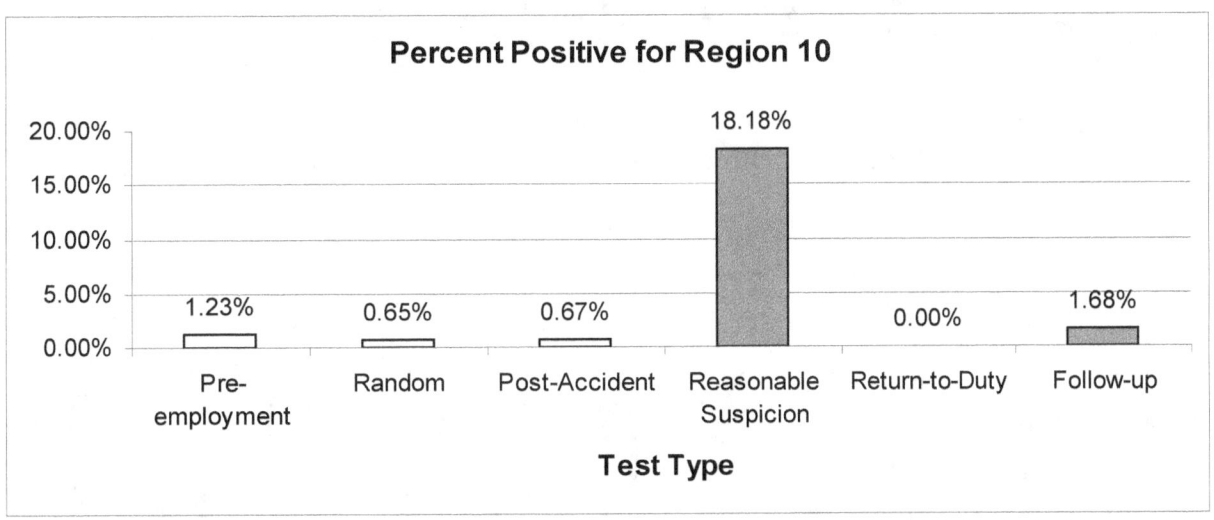

Figure 27. Percent Positive for All Test Types for Region 10

29

3.3.11 Drug Test Results for All Regions

Table 27 provides drug test results for all test types and drugs detected for each region. Figure 28 illustrates the percent positive for all test types by region.

Table 27. Drug Test Results for All Regions

| Region | Total Number of Test Results | Verified Negative Results | Verified Positive Results for One or More Drugs | Positive for Marijuana | Positive for Cocaine | Positive for PCP | Positive for Opiates | Positive for Amphetamines | Refusals | | | | Cancelled Tests |
									Adulterated	Substituted	"Shy Bladder" with No Medical Explanation	Other Refusals to Submit to Testing	
1	8,557	8,413	137	92	45	1	1	2	0	0	0	7	26
2	38,504	37,948	531	343	176	7	13	3	7	2	0	16	43
3	25,518	24,881	570	376	151	42	15	4	2	0	4	61	65
4	27,369	26,930	397	260	134	4	16	5	6	4	6	26	78
5	29,444	28,978	419	274	135	2	12	3	9	5	10	23	45
6	16,063	15,784	237	143	80	6	0	11	2	0	3	37	35
7	7,270	7,183	78	61	12	0	2	4	0	0	0	9	19
8	8,441	8,300	131	87	37	0	4	8	2	1	0	7	26
9	41,861	41,138	664	457	123	5	18	81	8	4	6	41	126
10	9,379	9,289	78	48	16	0	2	14	0	1	2	9	13
TOTAL	**212,406**	**208,844**	**3,242**	**2,141**	**909**	**67**	**83**	**135**	**36**	**17**	**31**	**236**	**476**

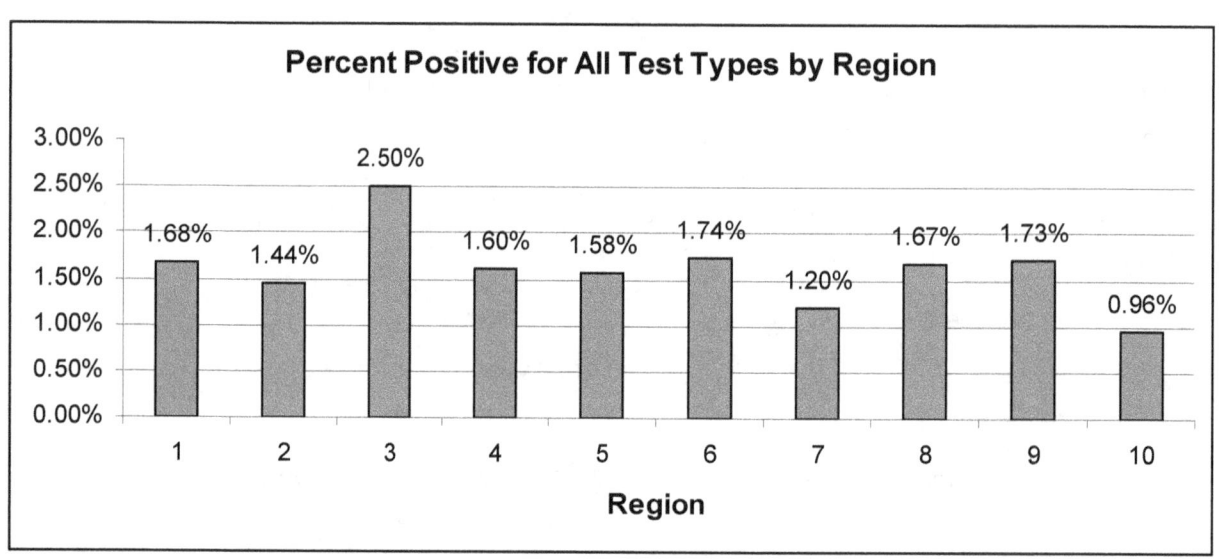

Figure 28. Percent Positive for All Test Types by Region

3.3.12 Drug Test Results for Transit Employers and Contractors

Table 28 provides drug test results for transit employers by region. Figure 29 illustrates the percent positive for transit employers by region. Table 29 provides drug test results for contractors by region. Figure 30 illustrates the percent positive for contractors by region.

Table 28. Drug Test Results for Transit Employers by Region

Region	Total Number of Test Results	Verified Negative Results	Verified Positive Results for One or More Drugs	Positive for Marijuana	Positive for Cocaine	Positive for PCP	Positive for Opiates	Positive for Amphetamines	Refusals				Cancelled Tests
									Adulterated	Substituted	"Shy Bladder" with No Medical Explanation	Other Refusals to Submit to Testing	
1	5,987	5,905	76	47	28	1	1	0	0	0	0	6	23
2	25,078	24,821	248	164	80	3	4	1	0	0	0	9	19
3	16,021	15,806	189	113	55	12	9	1	1	0	4	21	24
4	18,454	18,247	189	125	63	1	6	4	2	1	3	12	51
5	19,675	19,487	164	101	62	0	4	1	3	2	10	9	27
6	12,300	12,124	152	92	49	4	0	9	2	0	2	20	29
7	6,087	6,024	56	42	9	0	1	4	0	0	0	7	10
8	4,762	4,698	58	43	14	0	3	1	1	0	0	5	18
9	18,701	18,537	146	97	25	0	6	19	1	0	5	12	26
10	6,550	6,493	49	29	8	0	0	13	0	0	2	6	9
TOTAL	133,615	132,142	1,327	853	393	21	34	53	10	3	26	107	236

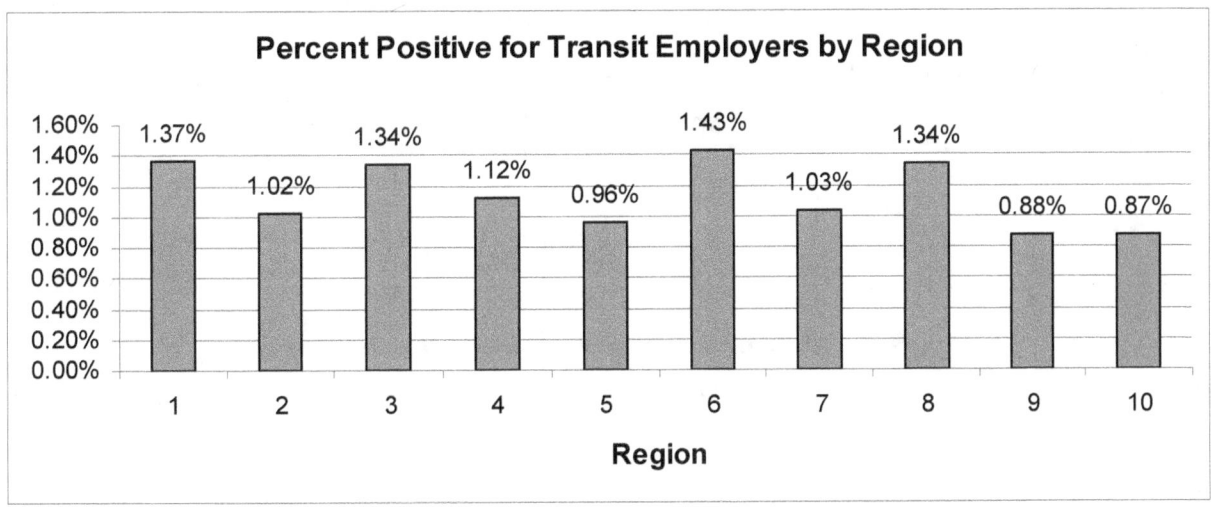

Figure 29. Percent Positive for Transit Employers by Region

31

Table 29. Drug Test Results for Contractors by Region

Region	Total Number of Test Results	Verified Negative Results	Verified Positive Results for One or More Drugs	Positive for Marijuana	Positive for Cocaine	Positive for PCP	Positive for Opiates	Positive for Amphetamines	Refusals				Cancelled Tests
									Adulterated	Substituted	"Shy Bladder" with No Medical Explanation	Other Refusals to Submit to Testing	
1	2,570	2,508	61	45	17	0	0	2	0	0	0	1	3
2	13,426	13,127	283	179	96	4	9	2	7	2	0	7	24
3	9,497	9,075	381	263	96	30	6	3	1	0	0	40	41
4	8,915	8,683	208	135	71	3	10	1	4	3	3	14	27
5	9,769	9,491	255	173	73	2	8	2	6	3	0	14	18
6	3,763	3,660	85	51	31	2	0	2	0	0	1	17	6
7	1,183	1,159	22	19	3	0	1	0	0	0	0	2	2
8	3,679	3,602	73	44	23	0	1	7	1	1	0	2	8
9	23,160	22,601	518	360	98	5	12	62	7	4	1	29	100
10	2,829	2,796	29	19	8	0	2	1	0	1	0	3	4
TOTAL	78,791	76,702	1,915	1,288	516	46	49	82	26	14	5	129	233

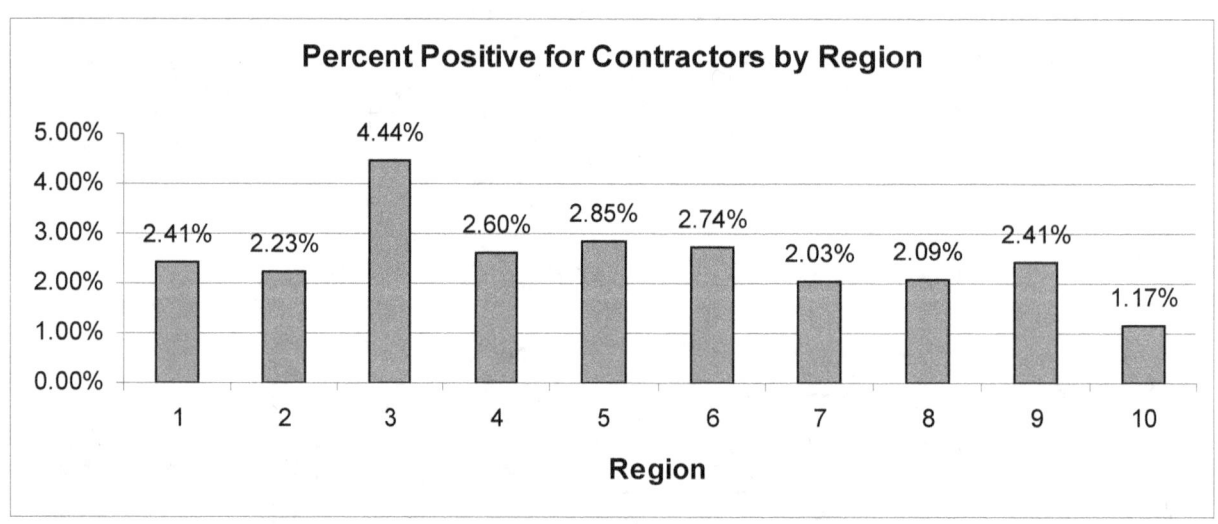

Figure 30. Percent Positive for Contractors by Region

4. Alcohol Test Results

4.1 Alcohol Test Results by Test Type and Employee Category

This section provides alcohol test results by test type conducted and for each employee category.

4.1.1 Pre-employment Alcohol Test Results

Table 30 provides alcohol results for pre-employment tests for each employee category. Figure 31 illustrates the percent positive for pre-employment tests by employee category.

Table 30. Pre-employment Alcohol Test Results by Employee Category

Employee Category	Total Number of Screening Test Results	Screening Tests with Results Below 0.02	Screening Tests with Results 0.02 or Greater	Number of Confirmation Test Results	Confirmation Tests with Results 0.02 to 0.039	Confirmation Tests with Results 0.04 or Greater	"Shy Lung" with No Medical Explanation	Other Refusals to Submit to Testing	Cancelled Tests
Revenue Vehicle Operation	11,203	11,187	16	16	3	9	0	0	1
Revenue Vehicle & Equipment Maintenance	1,298	1,296	2	2	0	2	0	0	1
Revenue Vehicle Control/Dispatch	410	409	1	1	0	1	0	0	0
CDL/Non-Revenue Vehicle	204	196	8	0	0	0	0	0	0
Armed Security Personnel	330	329	1	1	0	0	0	0	0
TOTAL	13,445	13,417	28	20	3	12	0	0	2

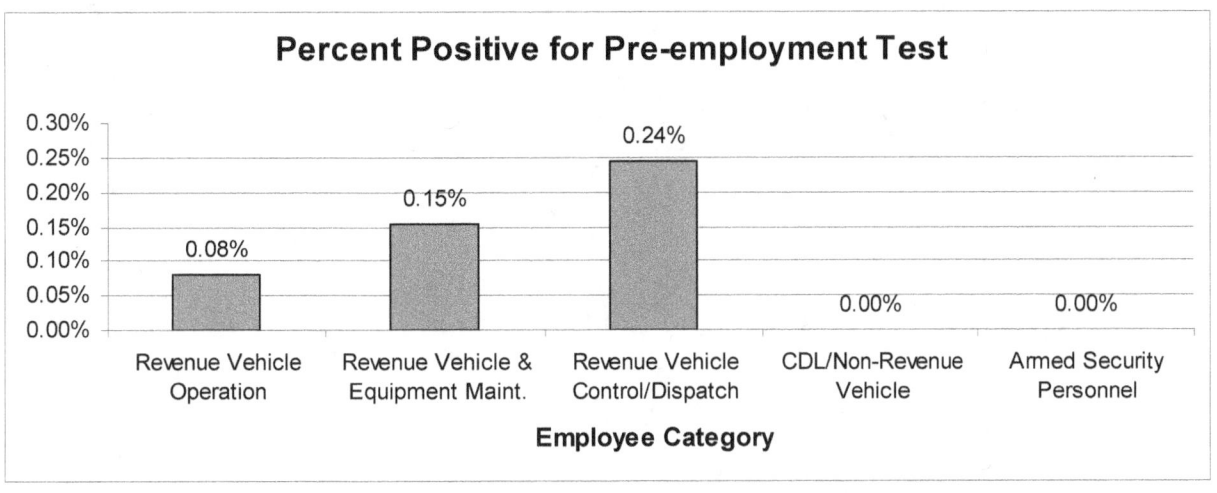

Figure 31. Percent Positive for Pre-employment Tests by Employee Category

4.1.2 Random Alcohol Test Results

Table 31 provides alcohol results for random tests for each employee category. Figure 32 illustrates the percent positive for random alcohol tests by employee category.

Table 31. Random Alcohol Test Results by Employee Category

Employee Category	Total Number of Screening Test Results	Screening Tests with Results Below 0.02	Screening Tests with Results 0.02 or Greater	Number of Confirmation Test Results	Confirmation Tests with Results 0.02 to 0.039	Confirmation Tests with Results 0.04 or Greater	"Shy Lung" with No Medical Explanation	Other Refusals to Submit to Testing	Cancelled Tests
Revenue Vehicle Operation	26,480	26,411	55	46	17	25	8	6	20
Revenue Vehicle & Equipment Maintenance	7,223	7,192	30	27	10	14	1	0	2
Revenue Vehicle Control/Dispatch	2,936	2,929	7	5	1	3	0	0	2
CDL/Non-Revenue Vehicle	682	680	2	1	0	0	0	0	4
Armed Security Personnel	735	735	0	0	0	0	0	0	0
Ferry Boat Operator	436	435	1	1	0	1	0	0	3
TOTAL	**38,492**	**38,382**	**95**	**80**	**28**	**43**	**9**	**6**	**31**

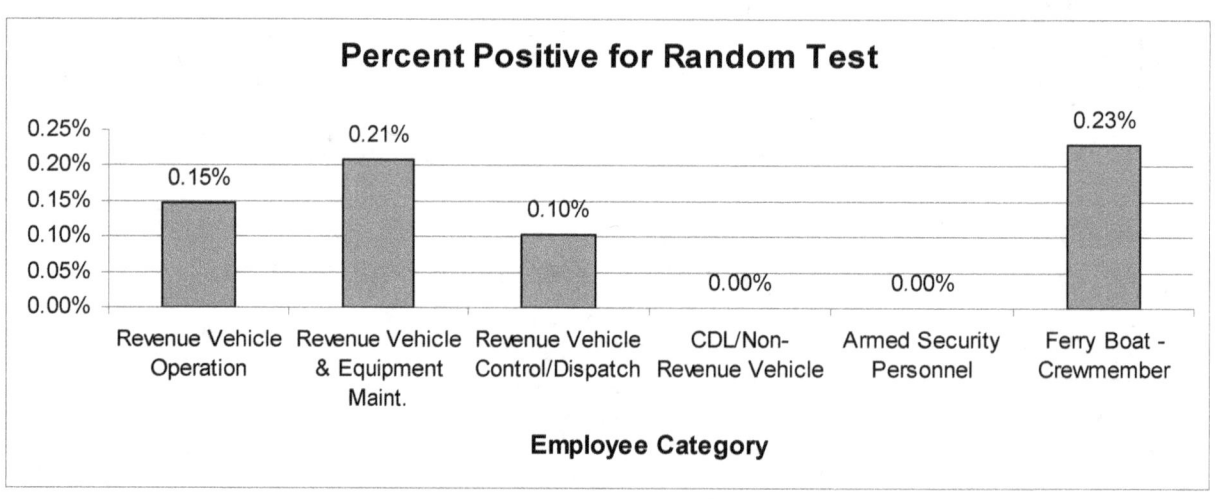

Figure 32. Percent Positive for Random Tests by Employee Category

4.1.3 Post-Accident Alcohol Test Results

Table 32 provides alcohol results for post-accident tests for each employee category. Figure 33 illustrates the percent positive for post-accident tests by employee category.

Table 32. Post-Accident Alcohol Test Results by Employee Category

Employee Category	Total Number of Screening Test Results	Screening Tests with Results Below 0.02	Screening Tests with Results 0.02 or Greater	Number of Confirmation Test Results	Confirmation Tests with Results 0.02 to 0.039	Confirmation Tests with Results 0.04 or Greater	"Shy Lung" with No Medical Explanation	Other Refusals to Submit to Testing	Cancelled Tests
Revenue Vehicle Operation	11,512	11,492	16	16	5	10	1	3	3
Revenue Vehicle & Equipment Maintenance	481	477	4	4	2	2	0	0	0
Revenue Vehicle Control/Dispatch	117	117	0	0	0	0	0	0	0
CDL/Non-Revenue Vehicle	56	55	1	0	0	0	0	0	0
Armed Security Personnel	80	80	0	0	0	0	0	0	0
TOTAL	**12,246**	**12,221**	**21**	**20**	**7**	**12**	**1**	**3**	**3**

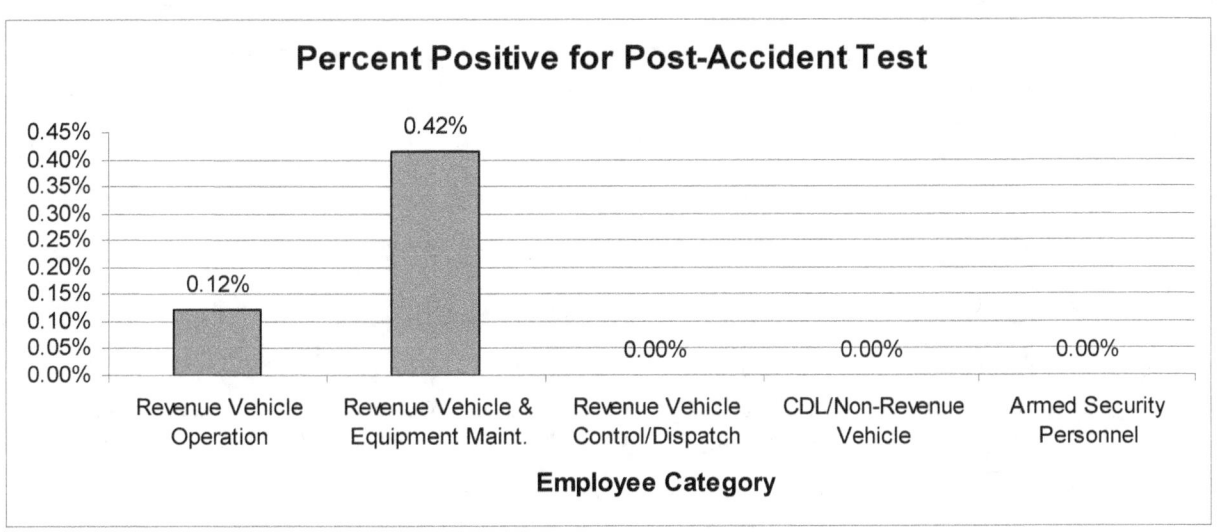

Figure 33. Percent Positive for Post-Accident Tests by Employee Category

4.1.4 Reasonable Suspicion Alcohol Test Results

Table 33 provides alcohol results for reasonable suspicion tests for each employee category. Figure 34 illustrates the percent positive for reasonable suspicion tests by employee category.

Table 33. Reasonable Suspicion Alcohol Test Results by Employee Category

Employee Category	Total Number of Screening Test Results	Screening Tests with Results Below 0.02	Screening Tests with Results 0.02 or Greater	Number of Confirmation Test Results	Confirmation Tests with Results 0.02 to 0.039	Confirmation Tests with Results 0.04 or Greater	"Shy Lung" with No Medical Explanation	Other Refusals to Submit to Testing	Cancelled Tests
Revenue Vehicle Operation	399	296	95	94	21	65	1	7	0
Revenue Vehicle & Equipment Maintenance	78	52	26	26	6	20	0	0	0
Revenue Vehicle Control/Dispatch	17	15	2	2	0	2	0	0	0
CDL/Non-Revenue Vehicle	6	4	2	1	0	1	0	0	2
Armed Security Personnel	3	3	0	0	0	0	0	0	0
TOTAL	**503**	**370**	**125**	**123**	**27**	**88**	**1**	**7**	**2**

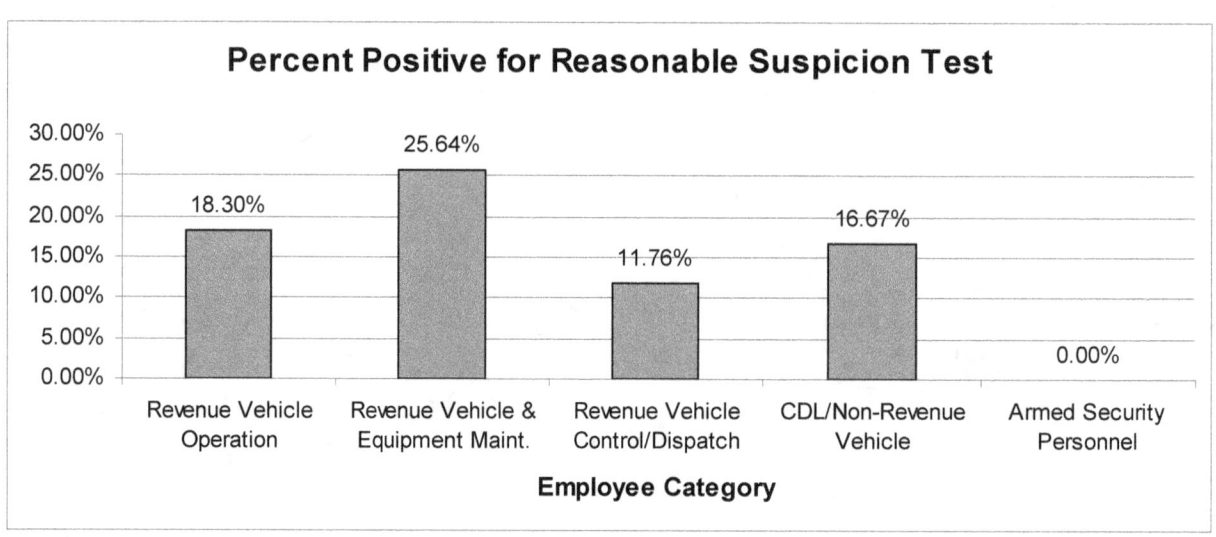

Figure 34. Percent Positive for Reasonable Suspicion Tests by Employee Category

36

4.1.5 Return-to-Duty Alcohol Test Results

Table 34 provides alcohol results for return-to-duty tests for each employee category. Figure 35 illustrates the percent positive for return-to-duty tests by employee category.

Table 34. Return-to-Duty Alcohol Test Results by Employee Category

Employee Category	Total Number of Screening Test Results	Screening Tests with Results Below 0.02	Screening Tests with Results 0.02 or Greater	Number of Confirmation Test Results	Confirmation Tests with Results 0.02 to 0.039	Confirmation Tests with Results 0.04 or Greater	"Shy Lung" with No Medical Explanation	Other Refusals to Submit to Testing	Cancelled Tests
Revenue Vehicle Operation	323	322	1	1	0	1	0	0	0
Revenue Vehicle & Equipment Maintenance	100	100	0	0	0	0	0	0	0
Revenue Vehicle Control/Dispatch	29	29	0	0	0	0	0	0	0
CDL/Non-Revenue Vehicle	5	5	0	0	0	0	0	0	0
Armed Security Personnel	0	0	0	0	0	0	0	0	0
TOTAL	**457**	**456**	**1**	**1**	**0**	**1**	**0**	**0**	**0**

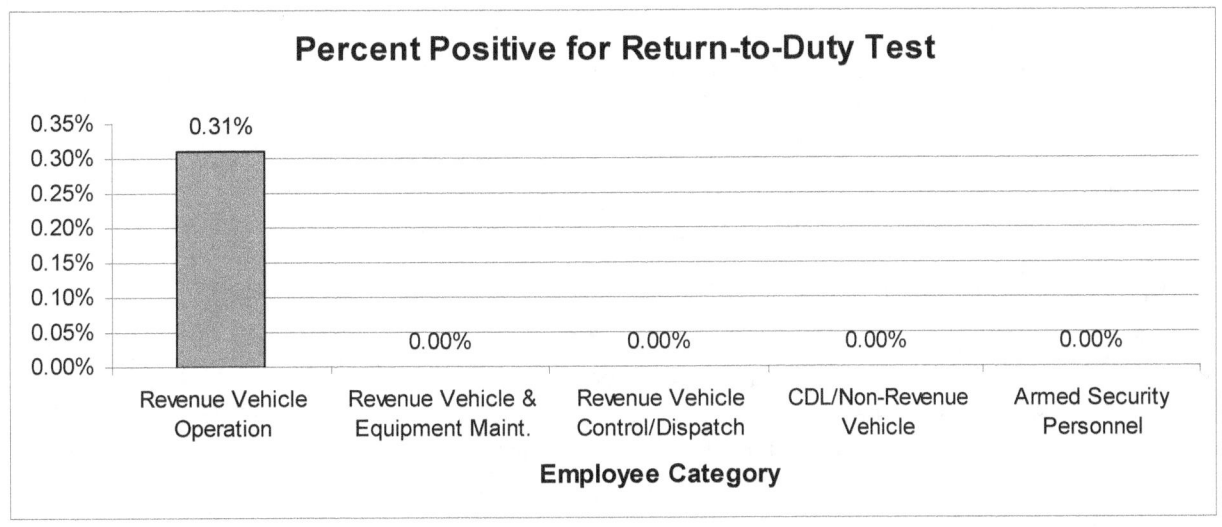

Figure 35. Percent Positive for Return-to-Duty Tests by Employee Category

37

4.1.6 Follow-up Alcohol Test Results

Table 35 provides alcohol results for follow-up tests for each employee category. Figure 36 illustrates the percent positive for follow-up tests by employee category.

Table 35. Follow-up Alcohol Test Results by Employee Category

Employee Category	Total Number of Screening Test Results	Screening Tests with Results Below 0.02	Screening Tests with Results 0.02 or Greater	Number of Confirmation Test Results	Confirmation Tests with Results 0.02 to 0.039	Confirmation Tests with Results 0.04 or Greater	"Shy Lung" with No Medical Explanation	Other Refusals to Submit to Testing	Cancelled Tests
Revenue Vehicle Operation	3,194	3,178	15	15	4	8	0	1	2
Revenue Vehicle & Equipment Maintenance	1,562	1,555	7	7	5	2	0	0	1
Revenue Vehicle Control/Dispatch	204	202	2	2	0	1	0	0	0
CDL/Non-Revenue Vehicle	114	114	0	0	0	0	0	0	0
Armed Security Personnel	32	32	0	0	0	0	0	0	0
TOTAL	5,106	5,081	24	24	9	11	0	1	3

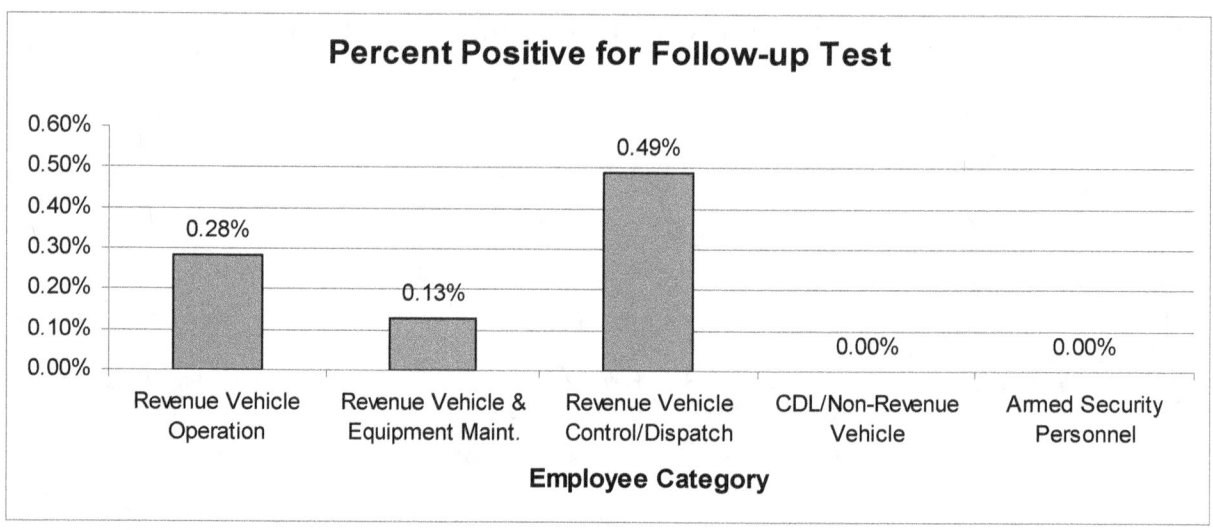

Figure 36. Percent Positive for Follow-up Tests by Employee Category

4.1.7 Alcohol Test Results for All Employee Categories by Test Type

Table 36 provides alcohol results for all employee categories by test type. Figure 37 illustrates the percent positive for all employee categories by test type.

Table 36. Alcohol Test Results for All Test Types

Employee Category	Total Number of Screening Test Results	Screening Tests with Results Below 0.02	Screening Tests with Results 0.02 or Greater	Number of Confirmation Test Results	Confirmation Tests with Results 0.02 to 0.039	Confirmation Tests with Results 0.04 or Greater	"Shy Lung" with No Medical Explanation	Other Refusals to Submit to Testing	Cancelled Tests
Pre-employment	13,445	13,417	28	20	3	12	0	0	2
Random	38,492	38,382	95	80	28	43	9	6	31
Post-Accident	12,246	12,221	21	20	7	12	1	3	3
Reasonable Suspicion	503	370	125	123	27	88	1	7	2
Return-to-Duty	457	456	1	1	0	1	0	0	0
Follow-up	5,106	5,081	24	24	9	11	0	1	3
TOTAL	**70,249**	**69,927**	**294**	**268**	**74**	**167**	**11**	**17**	**41**

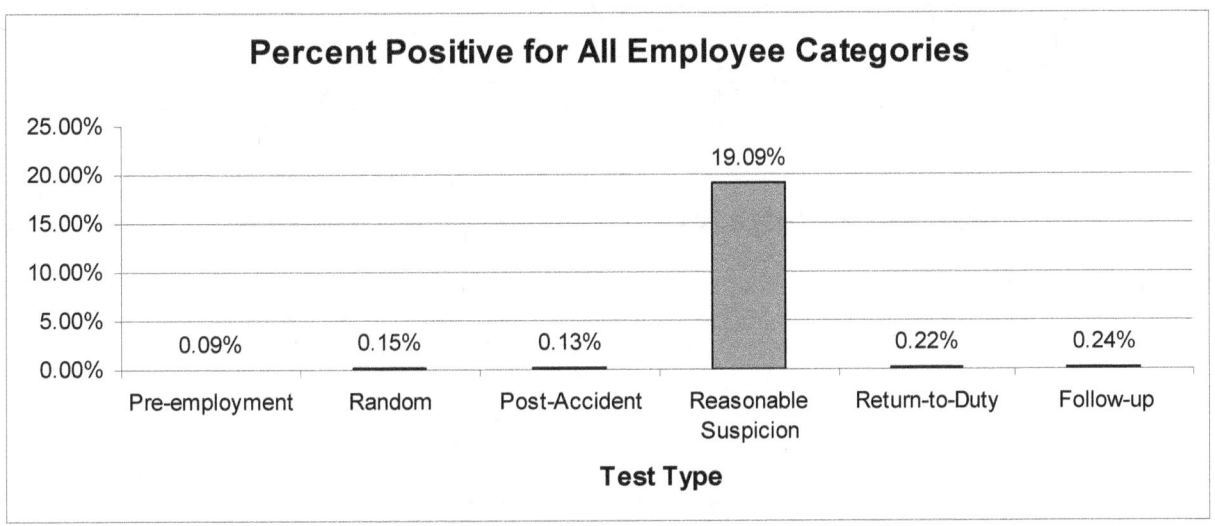

Figure 37. Percent Positive for All Employee Categories by Test Type

39

4.2 Alcohol Results by Employee Category

This section provides alcohol test results for each employee category by type of test conducted.

4.2.1 Revenue Vehicle Operation

Table 37 provides alcohol results for the revenue vehicle operation employee category by test type. Figure 38 illustrates the percent positive for the revenue vehicle operation employee category by test type.

Table 37. Alcohol Results for Revenue Vehicle Operation by Test Type

Test Type	Total Number of Screening Test Results	Screening Tests with Results Below 0.02	Screening Tests with Results 0.02 or Greater	Number of Confirmation Test Results	Confirmation Tests with Results 0.02 to 0.039	Confirmation Tests with Results 0.04 or Greater	"Shy Lung" with No Medical Explanation	Other Refusals to Submit to Testing	Cancelled Tests
Pre-employment	11,203	11,187	16	16	3	9	0	0	1
Random	26,480	26,411	55	46	17	25	8	6	20
Post-Accident	11,512	11,492	16	16	5	10	1	3	3
Reasonable Suspicion	399	296	95	94	21	65	1	7	0
Return-to-Duty	323	322	1	1	0	1	0	0	0
Follow-up	3,194	3,178	15	15	4	8	0	1	2
TOTAL	**53,111**	**52,886**	**198**	**188**	**50**	**118**	**10**	**17**	**26**

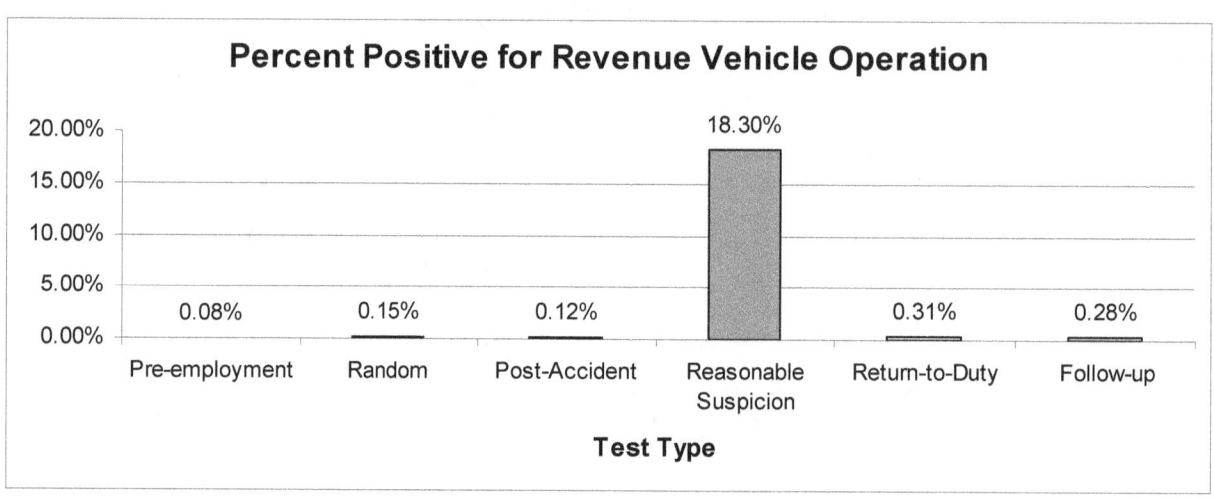

Figure 38. Percent Positive for the Revenue Vehicle Operation Employee Category by Test Type

40

4.2.2 Revenue Vehicle and Equipment Maintenance

Table 38 provides alcohol results for the revenue vehicle and equipment maintenance employee category by test type. Figure 39 illustrates the percent positive for the revenue vehicle and equipment maintenance employee category by test type.

Table 38. Alcohol Results for Revenue Vehicle and Equipment Maintenance by Test Type

Test Type	Total Number of Screening Test Results	Screening Tests with Results Below 0.02	Screening Tests with Results 0.02 or Greater	Number of Confirmation Test Results	Confirmation Tests with Results 0.02 to 0.039	Confirmation Tests with Results 0.04 or Greater	"Shy Lung" with No Medical Explanation	Other Refusals to Submit to Testing	Cancelled Tests
Pre-employment	1,298	1,296	2	2	0	2	0	0	1
Random	7,223	7,192	30	27	10	14	1	0	2
Post-Accident	481	477	4	4	2	2	0	0	0
Reasonable Suspicion	78	52	26	26	6	20	0	0	0
Return-to-Duty	100	100	0	0	0	0	0	0	0
Follow-up	1,562	1,555	7	7	5	2	0	0	1
TOTAL	**10,742**	**10,672**	**69**	**66**	**23**	**40**	**1**	**0**	**4**

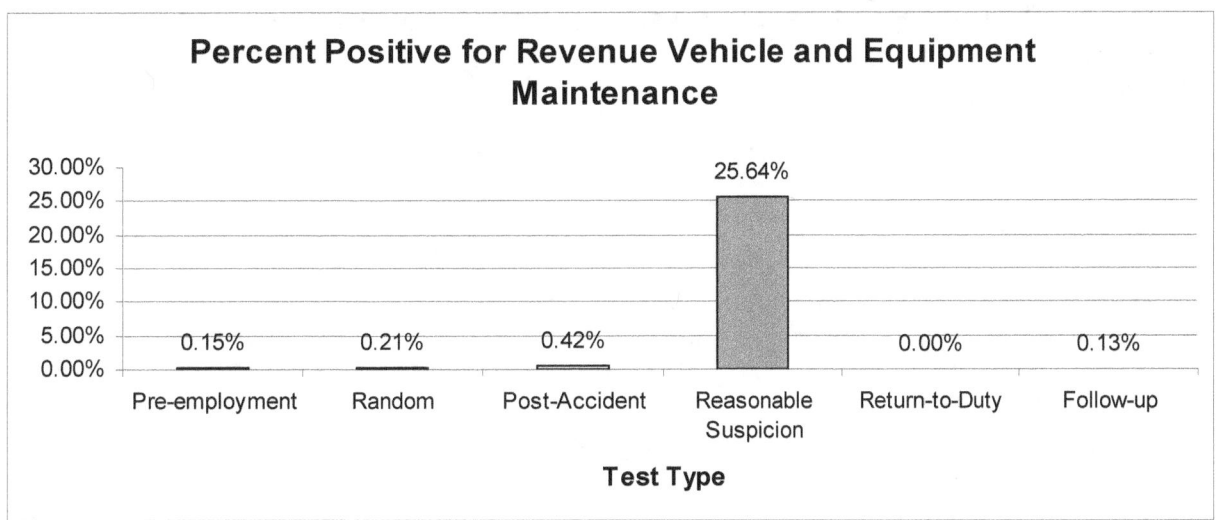

Figure 39. Percent Positive for the Revenue Vehicle and Equipment Maintenance Employee Category by Test Type

41

4.2.3 Revenue Vehicle Control/Dispatch

Table 39 provides alcohol results for the revenue vehicle control/dispatch employee category by test type. Figure 40 illustrates the percent positive for the revenue vehicle control/dispatch employee category by test type.

Table 39. Alcohol Results for Revenue Vehicle Control/Dispatch by Test Type

Test Type	Total Number of Screening Test Results	Screening Tests with Results Below 0.02	Screening Tests with Results 0.02 or Greater	Number of Confirmation Test Results	Confirmation Tests with Results 0.02 to 0.039	Confirmation Tests with Results 0.04 or Greater	"Shy Lung" with No Medical Explanation	Other Refusals to Submit to Testing	Cancelled Tests
Pre-employment	410	409	1	1	0	1	0	0	0
Random	2,936	2,929	7	5	1	3	0	0	2
Post-Accident	117	117	0	0	0	0	0	0	0
Reasonable Suspicion	17	15	2	2	0	2	0	0	0
Return-to-Duty	29	29	0	0	0	0	0	0	0
Follow-up	204	202	2	2	0	1	0	0	0
TOTAL	**3,713**	**3,701**	**12**	**10**	**1**	**7**	**0**	**0**	**2**

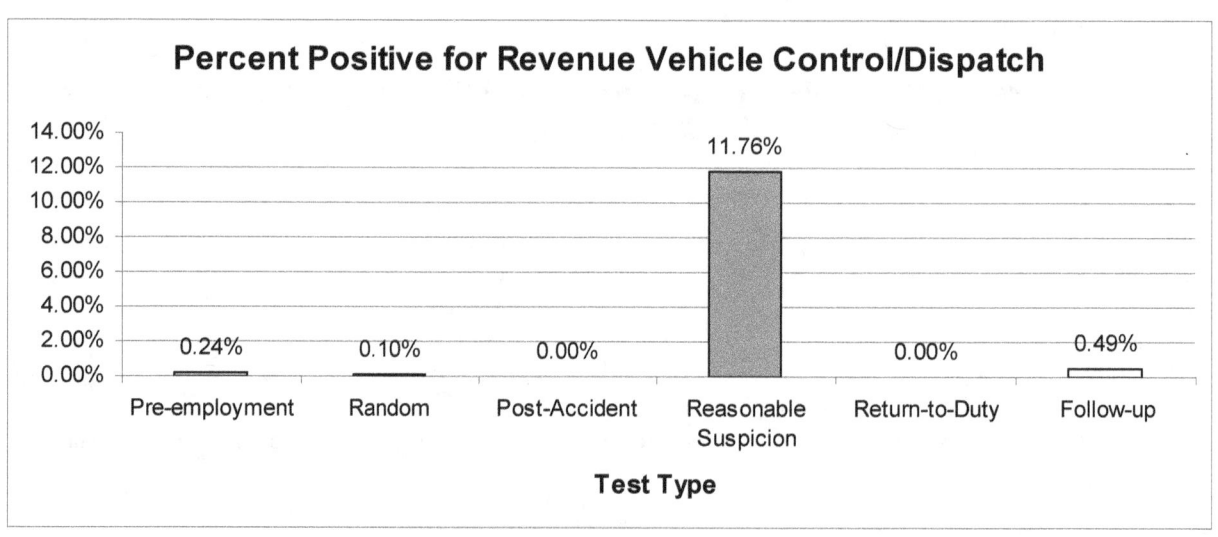

Figure 40. Percent Positive for the Revenue Vehicle Control/ Dispatch Employee Category by Test Type

4.2.4 CDL/Non-Revenue Vehicle

Table 40 provides alcohol results for the CDL/non-revenue vehicle employee category by test type. Figure 41 illustrates the percent positive for the CDL/non-revenue vehicle employee category by test type.

Table 40. Alcohol Results for CDL/Non-Revenue Vehicle by Test Type

Test Type	Total Number of Screening Test Results	Screening Tests with Results Below 0.02	Screening Tests with Results 0.02 or Greater	Number of Confirmation Test Results	Confirmation Tests with Results 0.02 to 0.039	Confirmation Tests with Results 0.04 or Greater	"Shy Lung" with No Medical Explanation	Other Refusals to Submit to Testing	Cancelled Tests
Pre-employment	204	196	8	0	0	0	0	0	0
Random	682	680	2	1	0	0	0	0	4
Post-Accident	56	55	1	0	0	0	0	0	0
Reasonable Suspicion	6	4	2	1	0	1	0	0	2
Return-to-Duty	5	5	0	0	0	0	0	0	0
Follow-up	114	114	0	0	0	0	0	0	0
TOTAL	**1,067**	**1,054**	**13**	**2**	**0**	**1**	**0**	**0**	**6**

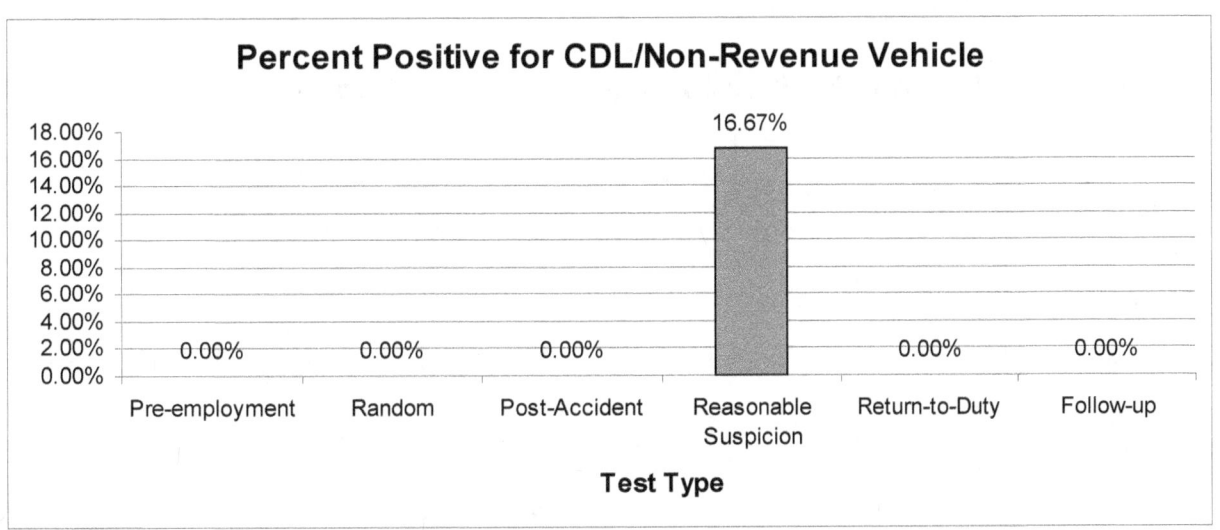

Figure 41. Percent Positive for the CDL/Non-Revenue Vehicle Employee Category by Test Type

43

4.2.5 Armed Security Personnel

Table 41 provides alcohol results for the armed security personnel employee category by test type. Figure 42 illustrates the percent positive for the armed security personnel employee category by test type.

Table 41. Alcohol Results for Armed Security Personnel by Test Type

Test Type	Total Number of Screening Test Results	Screening Tests with Results Below 0.02	Screening Tests with Results 0.02 or Greater	Number of Confirmation Test Results	Confirmation Tests with Results 0.02 to 0.039	Confirmation Tests with Results 0.04 or Greater	"Shy Lung" with No Medical Explanation	Other Refusals to Submit to Testing	Cancelled Tests
Pre-employment	330	329	1	1	0	0	0	0	0
Random	735	735	0	0	0	0	0	0	0
Post-Accident	80	80	0	0	0	0	0	0	0
Reasonable Suspicion	3	3	0	0	0	0	0	0	0
Return-to-Duty	0	0	0	0	0	0	0	0	0
Follow-up	32	32	0	0	0	0	0	0	0
TOTAL	**1,180**	**1,179**	**1**	**1**	**0**	**0**	**0**	**0**	**0**

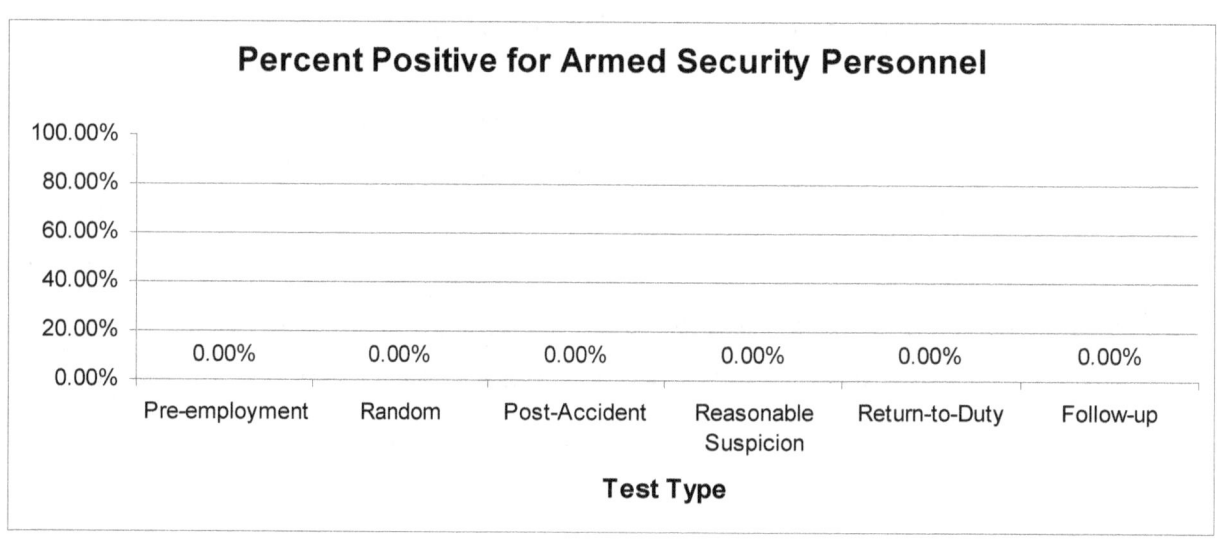

Figure 42. Percent Positive for the Armed Security Personnel Employee Category by Test Type

4.2.6　Ferry Boat Operator

On April 22, 2002, FTA published a Notice of Interpretation in the Federal Register that changed the applicability of the FTA Drug and Alcohol Testing Regulations to FTA-funded ferry boat operators. Previously, public transit ferry operators were required to comply with both the FTA and USCG regulations. The interpretation stated that FTA-funded ferry operations that comply with the relevant USCG drug and alcohol testing regulations were to be deemed in concurrent compliance with the FTA drug testing regulations. Since the USCG does not have a random alcohol testing provision that is similar to FTA's, the ferry operators were still required to comply with FTA's random alcohol testing requirements as defined in Section 655.45. On June 5, 2006, FTA published a Notice of Proposed Rulemaking (NPRM) that proposed to codify this interpretation in the final rule. If a ferry boat operator fails to be in compliance with the USCG testing regulations (46 CFR Part 4 and 16, and 33 CFR Part 95) or the FTA random alcohol testing regulations, the operator will be in non-compliance with 49 CFR Part 655. The employee is also subject to FTA consequences defined in Subpart G of the FTA regulations. The employer is responsible for the administrative and compliance certification requirements defined in Subparts H and I of the FTA regulations. This NPRM became a Final Rule, issued in November of 2006, and became effective January 2, 2007.

Table 42 provides alcohol results for the ferry boat operator employee category for random tests only. In 2007, the rate of ferry boat operators who tested positive for alcohol during a random test was 0.23 percent.

Table 42. Alcohol Results for Ferry Boat Operator for a Random Test

Test Type	Total Number of Screening Test Results	Screening Tests with Results Below 0.02	Screening Tests with Results 0.02 or Greater	Number of Confirmation Test Results	Confirmation Tests with Results 0.02 to 0.039	Confirmation Tests with Results 0.04 or Greater	"Shy Lung" with No Medical Explanation	Other Refusals to Submit to Testing	Cancelled Tests
Random	436	435	1	1	0	1	0	0	3
TOTAL	**436**	**435**	**1**	**1**	**0**	**1**	**0**	**0**	**3**

4.2.7 Alcohol Test Results for All Employee Categories

Table 43 provides alcohol results for all test types by employee category. Figure 43 illustrates the percent positive for all test types by employee category.

Table 43. Alcohol Results for All Employee Categories by Test Type

Employee Category	Total Number of Screening Test Results	Screening Tests with Results Below 0.02	Screening Tests with Results 0.02 or Greater	Number of Confirmation Test Results	Confirmation Tests with Results 0.02 to 0.039	Confirmation Tests with Results 0.04 or Greater	"Shy Lung" with No Medical Explanation	Other Refusals to Submit to Testing	Cancelled Tests
Revenue Vehicle Operation	53,111	52,886	198	188	50	118	10	17	26
Revenue Vehicle & Equipment Maintenance	10,742	10,672	69	66	23	40	1	0	4
Revenue Vehicle Control/Dispatch	3,713	3,701	12	10	1	7	0	0	2
CDL/Non-Revenue Vehicle	1,067	1,054	13	2	0	1	0	0	6
Armed Security Personnel	1,180	1,179	1	1	0	0	0	0	0
Ferry Boat Operator	436	435	1	1	0	1	0	0	3
TOTAL	**70,249**	**69,927**	**294**	**268**	**74**	**167**	**11**	**17**	**41**

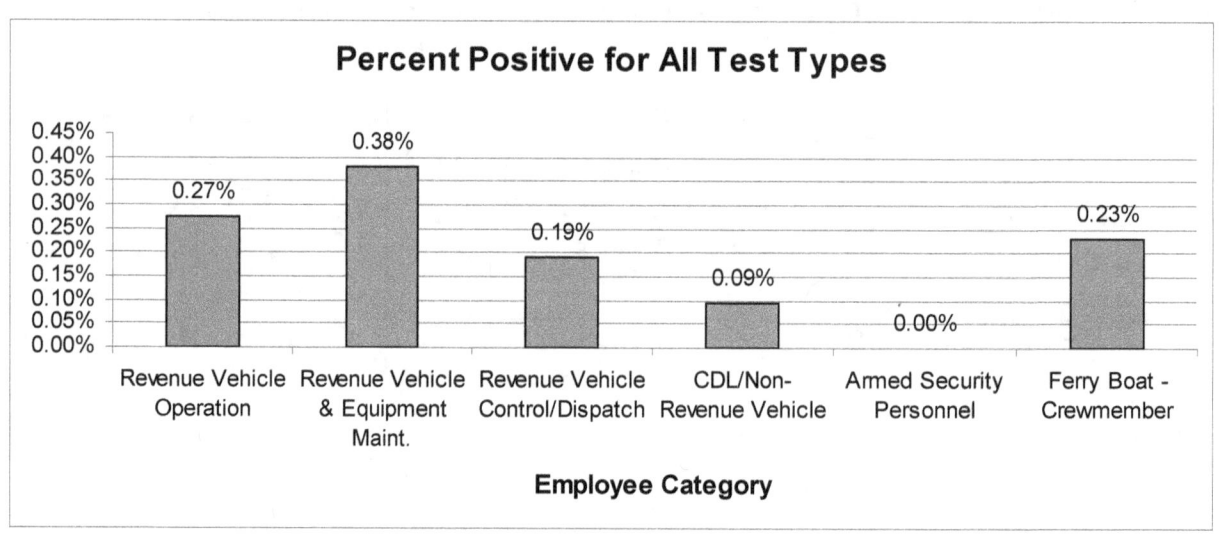

Figure 43. Percent Positive for All Test Types by Employee Category

46

4.3 Alcohol Test Results by Region

The following section provides alcohol test results for all test types, by each employee category, and for every region.

4.3.1 Alcohol Test Results for Region 1

Table 44 provides alcohol test results by employee category for all test types within Region 1. Figure 44 illustrates the percent positive by employee category for all test types within Region 1.

Table 44. Alcohol Results by Employee Category for All Test Types within Region 1

Employee Category	Total Number of Screening Test Results	Screening Tests with Results Below 0.02	Screening Tests with Results 0.02 or Greater	Number of Confirmation Test Results	Confirmation Tests with Results 0.02 to 0.039	Confirmation Tests with Results 0.04 or Greater	"Shy Lung" with No Medical Explanation	Other Refusals to Submit to Testing	Cancelled Tests
Revenue Vehicle Operation	1,823	1,810	13	13	2	10	0	0	0
Revenue Vehicle & Equipment Maintenance	329	328	1	1	0	1	0	0	0
Revenue Vehicle Control/Dispatch	125	125	0	0	0	0	0	0	0
CDL/Non-Revenue Vehicle	8	8	0	0	0	0	0	0	0
Armed Security Personnel	44	44	0	0	0	0	0	0	0
Ferry Boat Operator	4	4	0	0	0	0	0	0	0
TOTAL	**2,333**	**2,319**	**14**	**14**	**2**	**11**	**0**	**0**	**0**

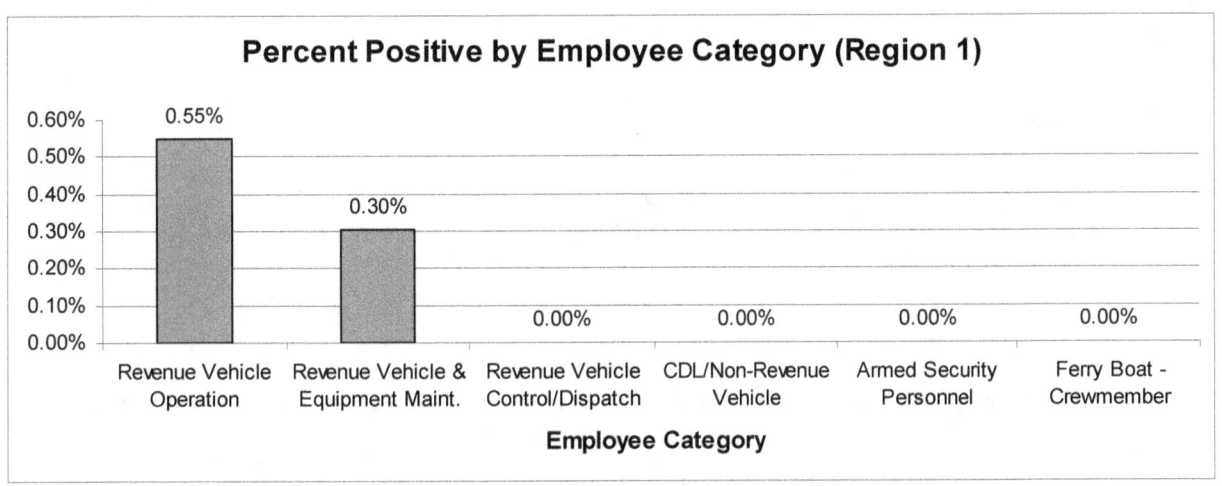

Figure 44. Percent Positive by Employee Category for All Test Types within Region 1

4.3.2 Alcohol Test Results for Region 2

Table 45 provides alcohol test results by employee category for all test types within Region 2. Figure 45 illustrates the percent positive by employee category for all test types within Region 2.

Table 45. Alcohol Results by Employee Category for All Test Types within Region 2

Employee Category	Total Number of Screening Test Results	Screening Tests with Results Below 0.02	Screening Tests with Results 0.02 or Greater	Number of Confirmation Test Results	Confirmation Tests with Results 0.02 to 0.039	Confirmation Tests with Results 0.04 or Greater	"Shy Lung" with No Medical Explanation	Other Refusals to Submit to Testing	Cancelled Tests
Revenue Vehicle Operation	9,655	9,628	24	24	6	15	3	0	1
Revenue Vehicle & Equipment Maintenance	2,943	2,928	15	15	8	6	0	0	1
Revenue Vehicle Control/Dispatch	748	743	5	5	0	5	0	0	0
CDL/Non-Revenue Vehicle	102	102	0	0	0	0	0	0	0
Armed Security Personnel	278	278	0	0	0	0	0	0	0
Ferry Boat Operator	425	424	1	1	0	1	0	0	3
TOTAL	14,151	14,103	45	45	14	27	3	0	5

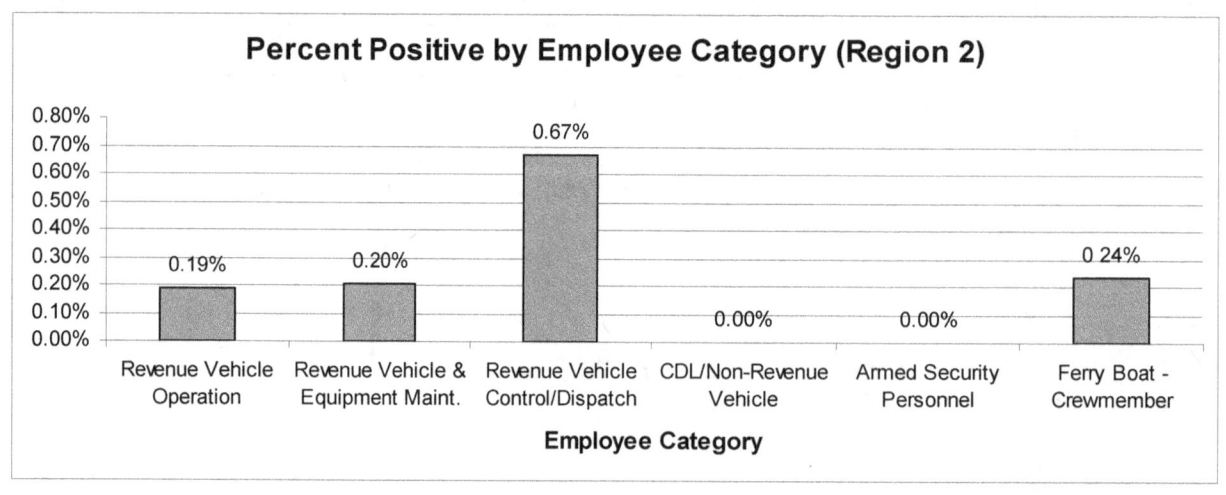

Figure 45. Percent Positive by Employee Category for All Test Types within Region 2

4.3.3 Alcohol Test Results for Region 3

Table 46 provides alcohol test results by employee category for all test types within Region 3. Figure 46 illustrates the percent positive by employee category for all test types within Region 3.

Table 46. Alcohol Results by Employee Category for All Test Types within Region 3

Employee Category	Total Number of Screening Test Results	Screening Tests with Results Below 0.02	Screening Tests with Results 0.02 or Greater	Number of Confirmation Test Results	Confirmation Tests with Results 0.02 to 0.039	Confirmation Tests with Results 0.04 or Greater	"Shy Lung" with No Medical Explanation	Other Refusals to Submit to Testing	Cancelled Tests
Revenue Vehicle Operation	9,272	9,240	29	28	4	21	1	2	2
Revenue Vehicle & Equipment Maintenance	1,976	1,960	16	16	6	9	0	0	0
Revenue Vehicle Control/Dispatch	367	367	0	0	0	0	0	0	0
CDL/Non-Revenue Vehicle	266	265	1	1	0	0	0	0	0
Armed Security Personnel	399	399	0	0	0	0	0	0	0
Ferry Boat Operator	0	0	0	0	0	0	0	0	0
TOTAL	**12,280**	**12,231**	**46**	**45**	**10**	**30**	**1**	**2**	**2**

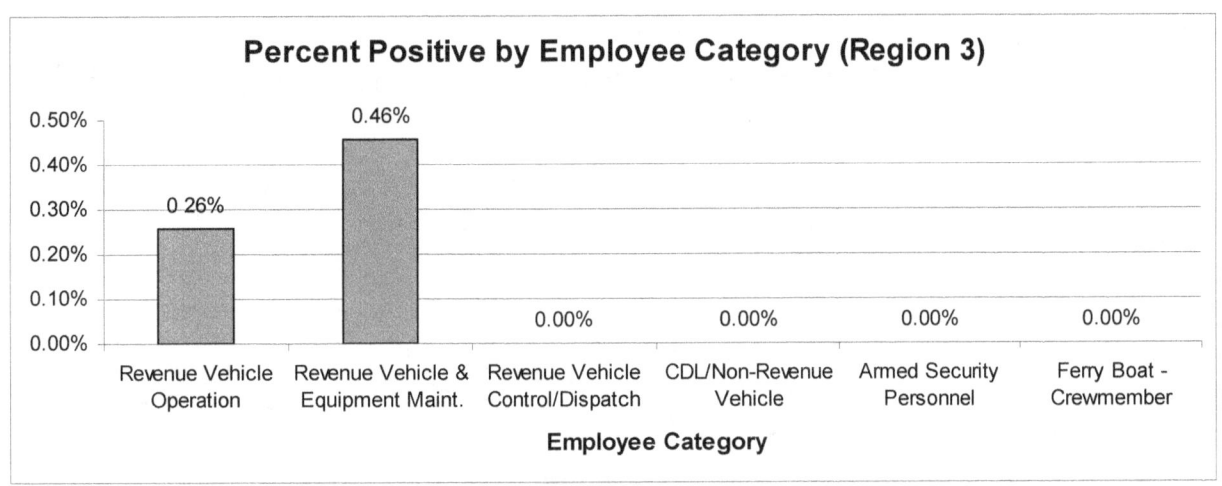

Figure 46. Percent Positive by Employee Category for All Test Types within Region 3

4.3.4 Alcohol Test Results for Region 4

Table 47 provides alcohol test results by employee category for all test types within Region 4. Figure 47 illustrates the percent positive by employee category for all test types within Region 4.

Table 47. Alcohol Results by Employee Category for All Test Types within Region 4

Employee Category	Total Number of Screening Test Results	Screening Tests with Results Below 0.02	Screening Tests with Results 0.02 or Greater	Number of Confirmation Test Results	Confirmation Tests with Results 0.02 to 0.039	Confirmation Tests with Results 0.04 or Greater	"Shy Lung" with No Medical Explanation	Other Refusals to Submit to Testing	Cancelled Tests
Revenue Vehicle Operation	6,150	6,137	8	8	1	5	1	4	2
Revenue Vehicle & Equipment Maintenance	1,184	1,179	5	5	0	4	0	0	0
Revenue Vehicle Control/Dispatch	711	707	4	3	1	0	0	0	0
CDL/Non-Revenue Vehicle	218	207	11	1	0	1	0	0	2
Armed Security Personnel	159	159	0	0	0	0	0	0	0
Ferry Boat Operator	1	1	0	0	0	0	0	0	0
TOTAL	**8,423**	**8,390**	**28**	**17**	**2**	**10**	**1**	**4**	**4**

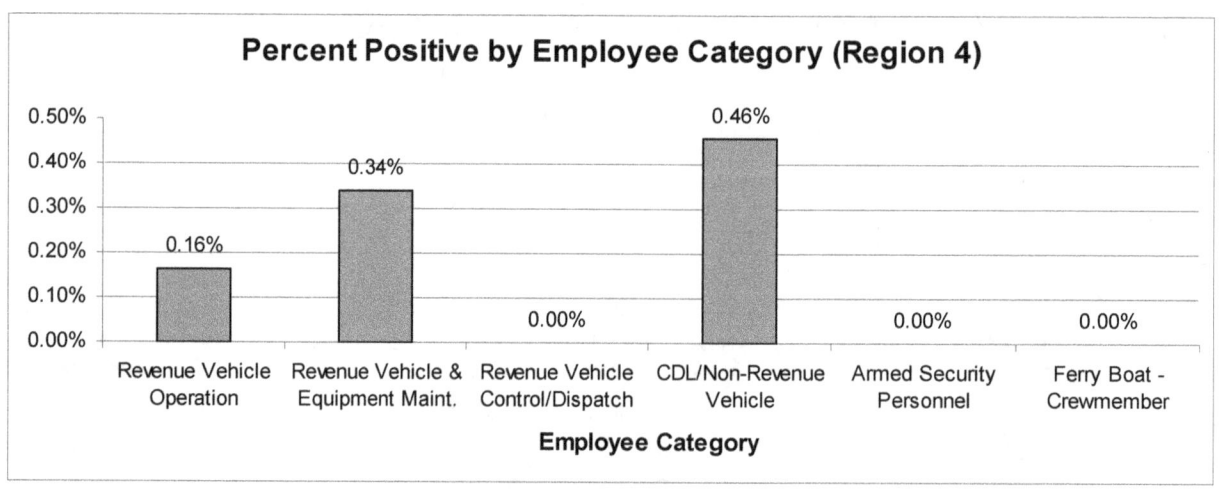

Figure 47. Percent Positive by Employee Category for All Test Types within Region 4

4.3.5 Alcohol Test Results for Region 5

Table 48 provides alcohol test results by employee category for all test types within Region 5. Figure 48 illustrates the percent positive by employee category for all test types within Region 5.

Table 48. Alcohol Results by Employee Category for All Test Types within Region 5

Employee Category	Total Number of Screening Test Results	Screening Tests with Results Below 0.02	Screening Tests with Results 0.02 or Greater	Number of Confirmation Test Results	Confirmation Tests with Results 0.02 to 0.039	Confirmation Tests with Results 0.04 or Greater	"Shy Lung" with No Medical Explanation	Other Refusals to Submit to Testing	Cancelled Tests
Revenue Vehicle Operation	8,073	8,030	38	38	11	24	1	4	7
Revenue Vehicle & Equipment Maintenance	1,345	1,336	8	8	3	5	1	0	1
Revenue Vehicle Control/Dispatch	546	544	2	2	0	2	0	0	1
CDL/Non-Revenue Vehicle	123	123	0	0	0	0	0	0	4
Armed Security Personnel	21	21	0	0	0	0	0	0	0
Ferry Boat Operator	0	0	0	0	0	0	0	0	0
TOTAL	10,108	10,054	48	48	14	31	2	4	13

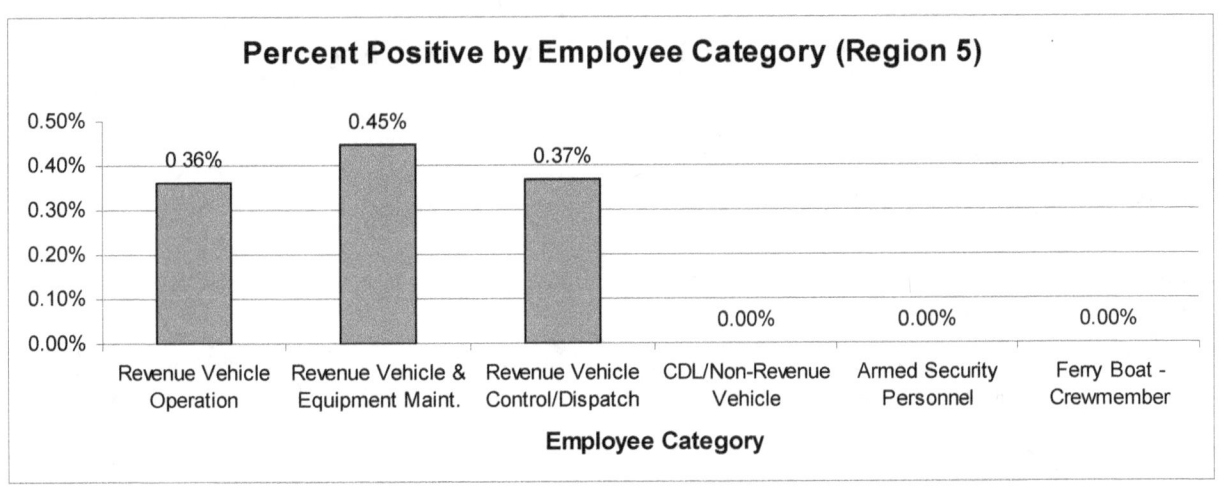

Figure 48. Percent Positive by Employee Category for All Test Types within Region 5

4.3.6 Alcohol Test Results for Region 6

Table 49 provides alcohol test results by employee category for all test types within Region 6. Figure 49 illustrates the percent positive by employee category for all test types within Region 6.

Table 49. Alcohol Results by Employee Category for All Test Types within Region 6

Employee Category	Total Number of Screening Test Results	Screening Tests with Results Below 0.02	Screening Tests with Results 0.02 or Greater	Number of Confirmation Test Results	Confirmation Tests with Results 0.02 to 0.039	Confirmation Tests with Results 0.04 or Greater	"Shy Lung" with No Medical Explanation	Other Refusals to Submit to Testing	Cancelled Tests
Revenue Vehicle Operation	3,501	3,481	19	19	7	11	0	1	3
Revenue Vehicle & Equipment Maintenance	644	641	3	3	1	2	0	0	0
Revenue Vehicle Control/Dispatch	296	296	0	0	0	0	0	0	0
CDL/Non-Revenue Vehicle	93	93	0	0	0	0	0	0	0
Armed Security Personnel	117	117	0	0	0	0	0	0	0
Ferry Boat Operator	0	0	0	0	0	0	0	0	0
TOTAL	4,651	4,628	22	22	8	13	0	1	3

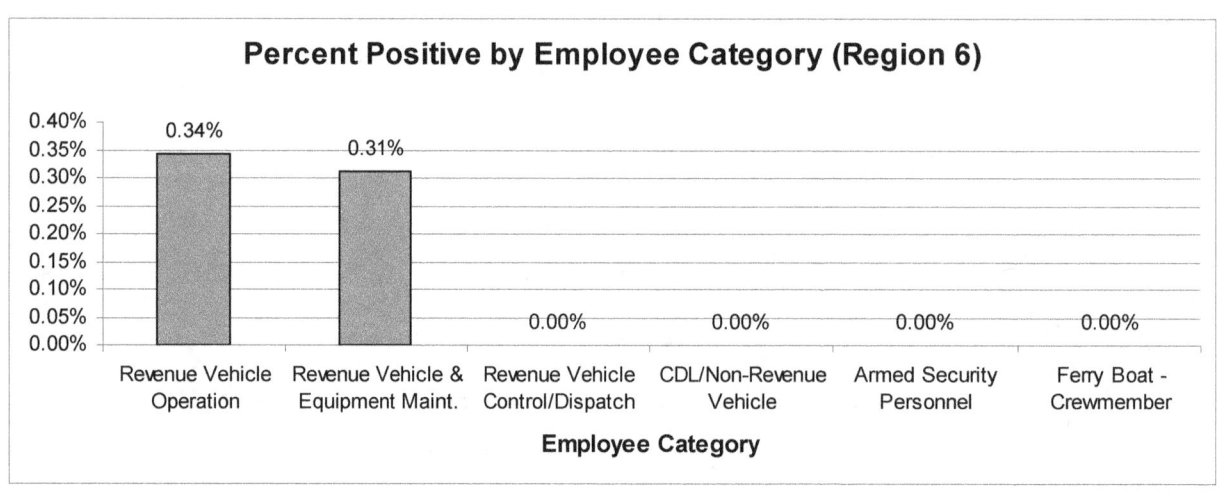

Figure 49. Percent Positive by Employee Category for All Test Types within Region 6

4.3.7   Alcohol Test Results for Region 7

Table 50 provides alcohol test results by employee category for all test types within Region 7. Figure 50 illustrates the percent positive by employee category for all test types within Region 7.

Table 50. Alcohol Results by Employee Category for All Test Types within Region 7

Employee Category	Total Number of Screening Test Results	Screening Tests with Results Below 0.02	Screening Tests with Results 0.02 or Greater	Number of Confirmation Test Results	Confirmation Tests with Results 0.02 to 0.039	Confirmation Tests with Results 0.04 or Greater	"Shy Lung" with No Medical Explanation	Other Refusals to Submit to Testing	Cancelled Tests
Revenue Vehicle Operation	1,601	1,590	9	9	3	5	1	1	2
Revenue Vehicle & Equipment Maintenance	190	190	0	0	0	0	0	0	0
Revenue Vehicle Control/Dispatch	71	71	0	0	0	0	0	0	0
CDL/Non-Revenue Vehicle	16	16	0	0	0	0	0	0	0
Armed Security Personnel	4	4	0	0	0	0	0	0	0
Ferry Boat Operator	0	0	0	0	0	0	0	0	0
TOTAL	1,882	1,871	9	9	3	5	1	1	2

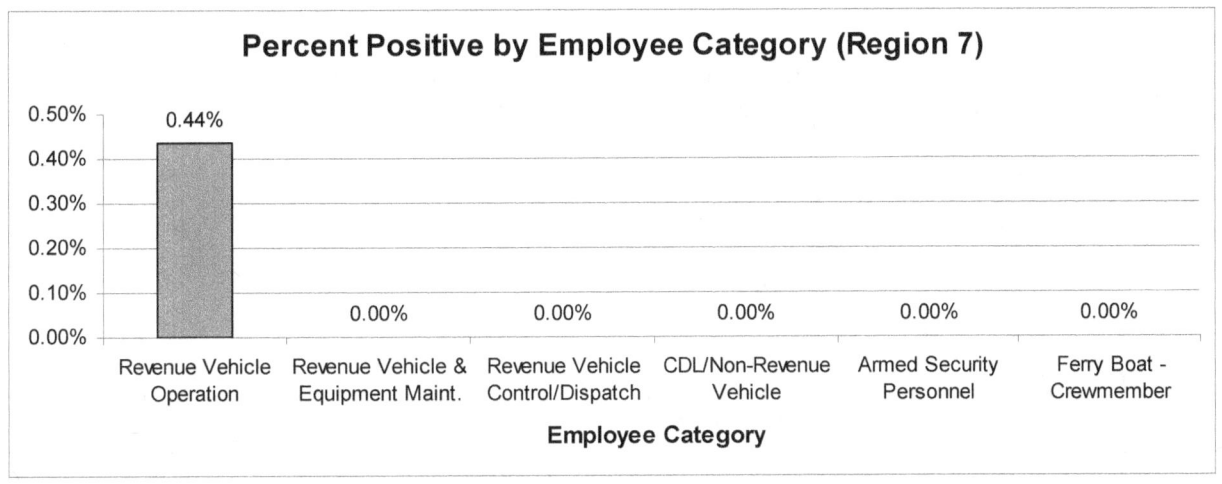

Figure 50. Percent Positive by Employee Category for All Test Types within Region 7

4.3.8 Alcohol Test Results for Region 8

Table 51 provides alcohol test results by employee category for all test types within Region 8. Figure 51 illustrates the percent positive by employee category for all test types within Region 8.

Table 51. Alcohol Results by Employee Category for All Test Types within Region 8

Employee Category	Total Number of Screening Test Results	Screening Tests with Results Below 0.02	Screening Tests with Results 0.02 or Greater	Number of Confirmation Test Results	Confirmation Tests with Results 0.02 to 0.039	Confirmation Tests with Results 0.04 or Greater	"Shy Lung" with No Medical Explanation	Other Refusals to Submit to Testing	Cancelled Tests
Revenue Vehicle Operation	1,170	1,148	20	11	3	5	0	2	0
Revenue Vehicle & Equipment Maintenance	177	173	4	1	0	1	0	0	0
Revenue Vehicle Control/Dispatch	120	119	1	0	0	0	0	0	0
CDL/Non-Revenue Vehicle	28	28	0	0	0	0	0	0	0
Armed Security Personnel	15	15	0	0	0	0	0	0	0
Ferry Boat Operator	0	0	0	0	0	0	0	0	0
TOTAL	1,510	1,483	25	12	3	6	0	2	0

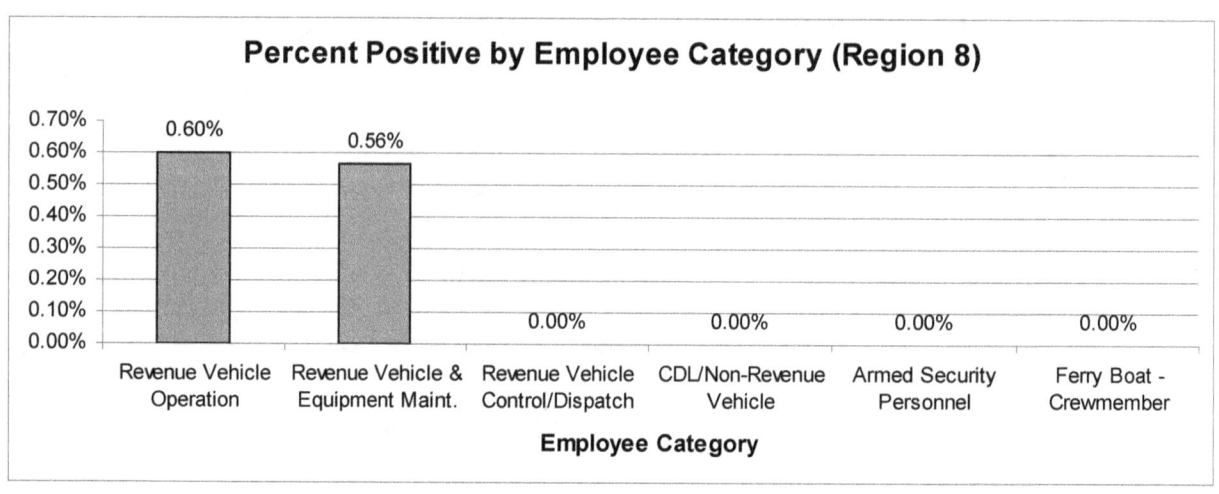

Figure 51. Percent Positive by Employee Category for All Test Types within Region 8

4.3.9 Alcohol Test Results for Region 9

Table 52 provides alcohol test results by employee category for all test types within Region 9. Figure 52 illustrates the percent positive by employee category for all test types within Region 9.

Table 52. Alcohol Results by Employee Category for All Test Types within Region 9

Employee Category	Total Number of Screening Test Results	Screening Tests with Results Below 0.02	Screening Tests with Results 0.02 or Greater	Number of Confirmation Test Results	Confirmation Tests with Results 0.02 to 0.039	Confirmation Tests with Results 0.04 or Greater	"Shy Lung" with No Medical Explanation	Other Refusals to Submit to Testing	Cancelled Tests
Revenue Vehicle Operation	9,647	9,611	31	31	10	18	2	3	6
Revenue Vehicle & Equipment Maintenance	1,660	1,644	16	16	5	11	0	0	2
Revenue Vehicle Control/Dispatch	570	570	0	0	0	0	0	0	0
CDL/Non-Revenue Vehicle	141	140	1	0	0	0	0	0	0
Armed Security Personnel	143	142	1	1	0	0	0	0	0
Ferry Boat Operator	6	6	0	0	0	0	0	0	0
TOTAL	12,167	12,113	49	48	15	29	2	3	8

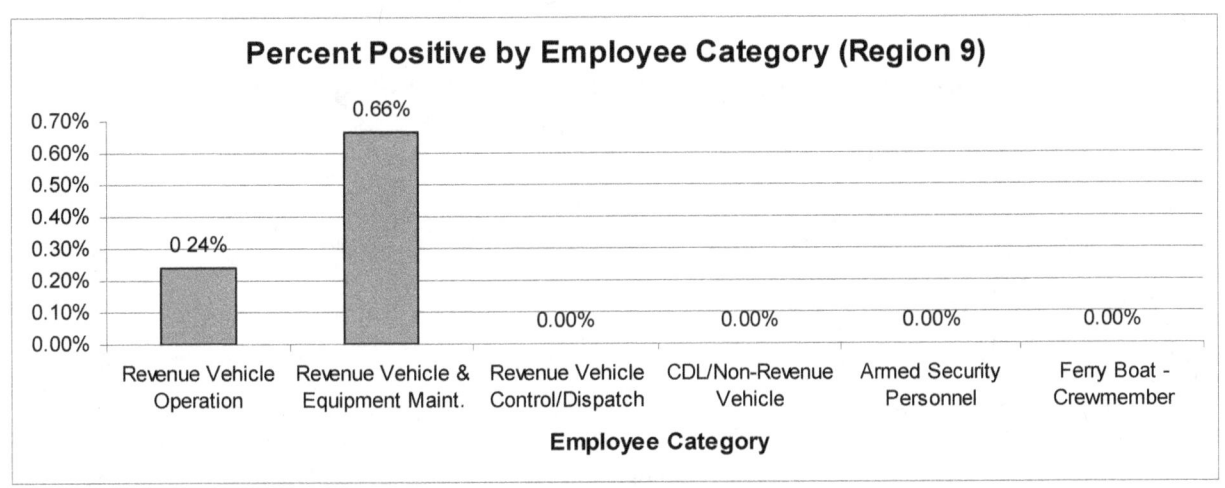

Figure 52. Percent Positive by Employee Category for All Test Types within Region 9

4.3.10 Alcohol Test Results for Region 10

Table 53 provides alcohol test results by employee category for all test types within Region 10. Figure 53 illustrates the percent positive by employee category for all test types within Region 10.

Table 53. Alcohol Results by Employee Category for All Test Types within Region 10

Employee Category	Total Number of Screening Test Results	Screening Tests with Results Below 0.02	Screening Tests with Results 0.02 or Greater	Number of Confirmation Test Results	Confirmation Tests with Results 0.02 to 0.039	Confirmation Tests with Results 0.04 or Greater	"Shy Lung" with No Medical Explanation	Other Refusals to Submit to Testing	Cancelled Tests
Revenue Vehicle Operation	2,202	2,195	6	6	3	3	1	0	3
Revenue Vehicle & Equipment Maintenance	294	293	1	1	0	1	0	0	0
Revenue Vehicle Control/Dispatch	158	158	0	0	0	0	0	0	1
CDL/Non-Revenue Vehicle	72	72	0	0	0	0	0	0	0
Armed Security Personnel	0	0	0	0	0	0	0	0	0
Ferry Boat Operator	0	0	0	0	0	0	0	0	0
TOTAL	2,726	2,718	7	7	3	4	1	0	4

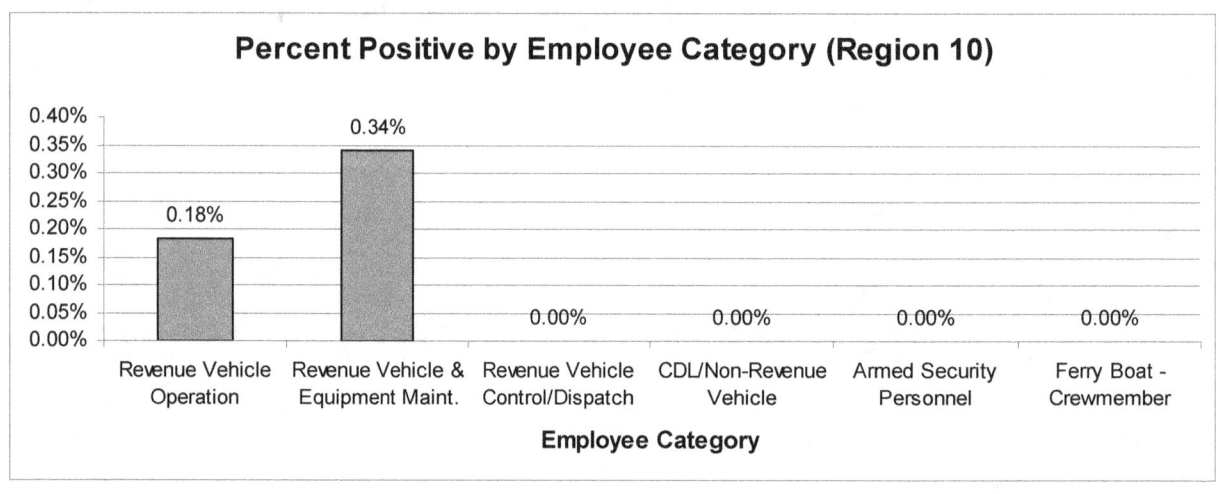

Figure 53. Percent Positive by Employee Category for All Test Types within Region 10

4.3.11 Alcohol Test Results for All Test Types by Region

Table 54 provides alcohol test results for all employee categories and test types for all of the regions. Figure 54 illustrates the percent positive for all employee categories and test types for each region.

Table 54. Alcohol Results for All Employee Categories and Test Types by Region

Region	Total Number of Screening Test Results	Screening Tests with Results Below 0.02	Screening Tests with Results 0.02 or Greater	Number of Confirmation Test Results	Confirmation Tests with Results 0.02 to 0.039	Confirmation Tests with Results 0.04 or Greater	"Shy Lung" with No Medical Explanation	Other Refusals to Submit to Testing	Cancelled Tests
1	2,333	2,319	14	14	2	11	0	0	0
2	14,151	14,103	45	45	14	27	3	0	5
3	12,280	12,231	46	45	10	30	1	2	2
4	8,423	8,390	28	17	2	10	1	4	4
5	10,108	10,054	48	48	14	31	2	4	13
6	4,651	4,628	22	22	8	13	0	1	3
7	1,882	1,871	9	9	3	5	1	1	2
8	1,510	1,483	25	12	3	6	0	2	0
9	12,167	12,113	49	48	15	29	2	3	8
10	2,726	2,718	7	7	3	4	1	0	4
TOTAL	70,231	69,910	293	267	74	166	11	17	41

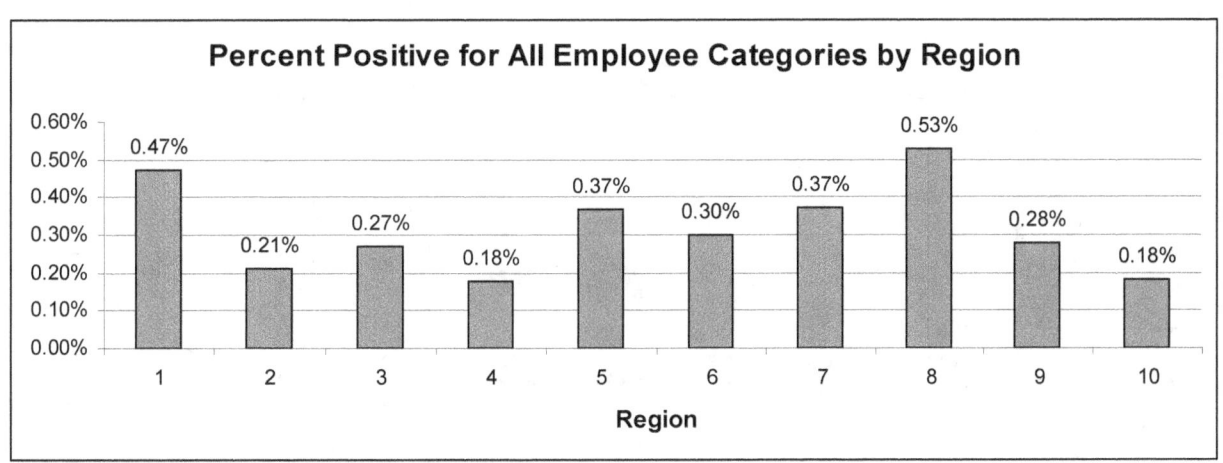

Figure 54. Percent Positive for All Employee Categories and Test Types by Region

4.4 Transit Employer and Contractor Alcohol Test Results

4.4.1 Alcohol Test Results for Transit Employers for All Test Types by Region

Table 55 provides alcohol test results for transit employers for all test types by region. Figure 55 illustrates the percent positive for transit employers for all test types by region.

Table 55. Alcohol Results for Transit Employers for All Test Types by Region

Region	Total Number of Screening Test Results	Screening Tests with Results Below 0.02	Screening Tests with Results 0.02 or Greater	Number of Confirmation Test Results	Confirmation Tests with Results 0.02 to 0.039	Confirmation Tests with Results 0.04 or Greater	"Shy Lung" with No Medical Explanation	Other Refusals to Submit to Testing	Cancelled Tests
1	1,757	1,747	10	10	0	10	0	0	0
2	10,584	10,554	29	29	11	15	1	0	4
3	9,338	9,303	34	33	6	23	1	0	2
4	6,795	6,769	23	12	1	8	0	3	4
5	6,886	6,844	39	39	13	24	2	1	12
6	3,912	3,891	20	20	6	13	0	1	1
7	1,578	1,568	8	8	3	5	1	1	2
8	1,078	1,058	18	5	1	4	0	2	0
9	8,278	8,258	18	18	6	12	0	2	4
10	2,223	2,218	5	5	3	2	0	0	2
TOTAL	52,429	52,210	204	179	50	116	5	10	31

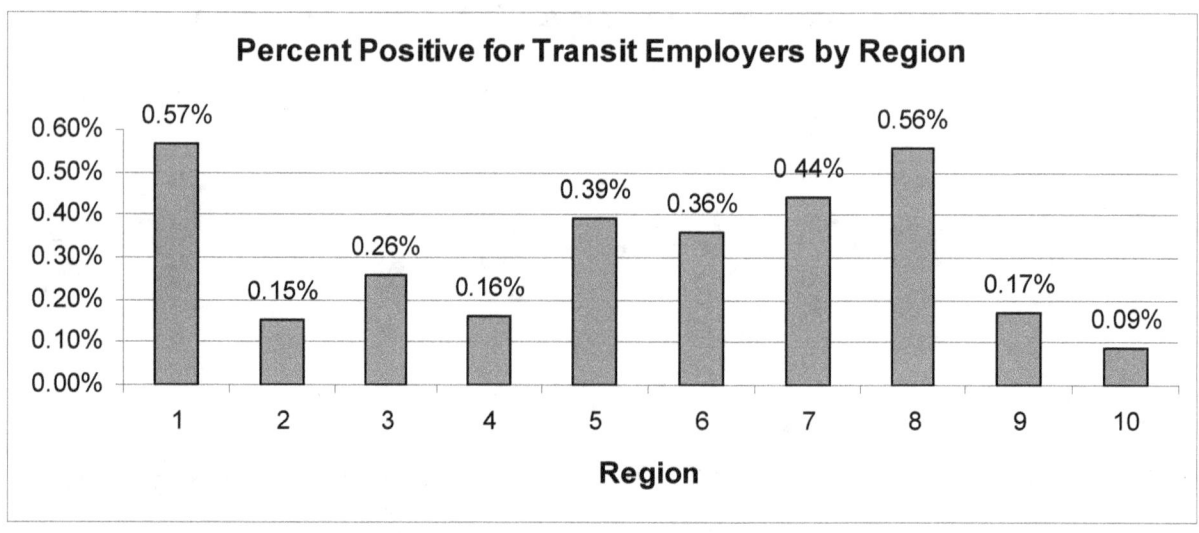

Figure 55. Percent Positive for Transit Employers for All Test Types by Region

4.4.2 Alcohol Test Results for Contractors for All Test Types by Region

Table 56 provides alcohol test results for contractors for all test types by region. Figure 56 illustrates the percent positive for contractors for all test types by region.

Table 56. Alcohol Results for Contractors for All Test Types by Region

Region	Total Number of Screening Test Results	Screening Tests with Results Below 0.02	Screening Tests with Results 0.02 or Greater	Number of Confirmation Test Results	Confirmation Tests with Results 0.02 to 0.039	Confirmation Tests with Results 0.04 or Greater	"Shy Lung" with No Medical Explanation	Other Refusals to Submit to Testing	Cancelled Tests
1	576	572	4	4	2	1	0	0	0
2	3,567	3,549	16	16	3	12	2	0	1
3	2,942	2,928	12	12	4	7	0	2	0
4	1,628	1,621	5	5	1	2	1	1	0
5	3,222	3,210	9	9	1	7	0	3	1
6	739	737	2	2	2	0	0	0	2
7	304	303	1	1	0	0	0	0	0
8	432	425	7	7	2	2	0	0	0
9	3,889	3,855	31	30	9	17	2	1	4
10	503	500	2	2	0	2	1	0	2
TOTAL	17,802	17,700	89	88	24	50	6	7	10

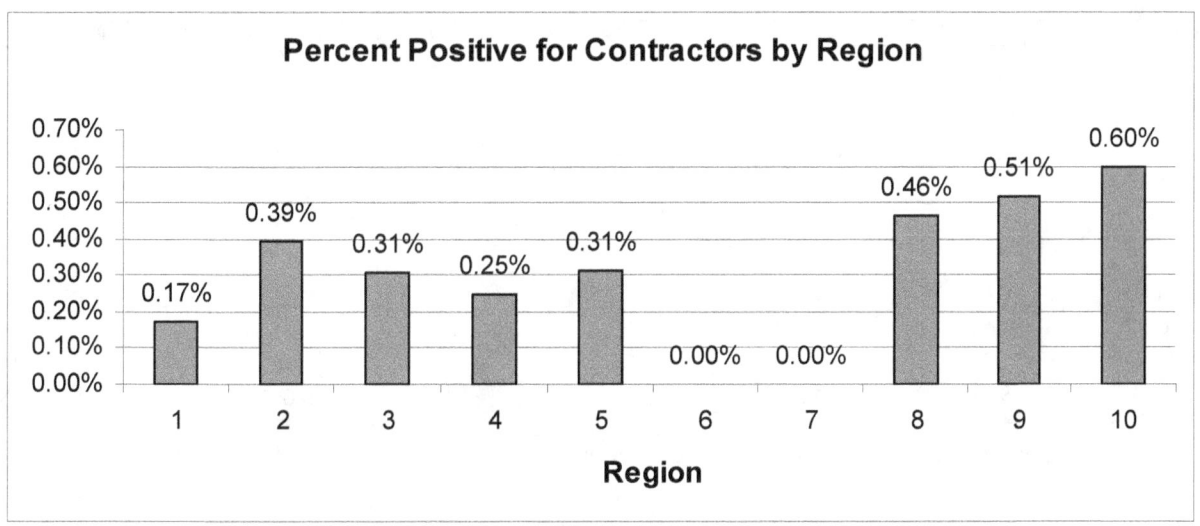

Figure 56. Percent Positive for Contractors for All Test Types by Region

4.5 Alcohol Test Results by Test Type for Each Region

This section provides alcohol test results by test type for all employee categories within each region.

4.5.1 Alcohol Test Results for Region 1

Table 57 provides alcohol test results for all employee categories by test type within Region 1. Figure 57 illustrates the percent positive for all employee categories by test type within Region 1.

Table 57. Alcohol Results for All Employee Categories by Test Type for Region 1

Test Type	Total Number of Screening Test Results	Screening Tests with Results Below 0.02	Screening Tests with Results 0.02 or Greater	Number of Confirmation Test Results	Confirmation Tests with Results 0.02 to 0.039	Confirmation Tests with Results 0.04 or Greater	"Shy Lung" with No Medical Explanation	Other Refusals to Submit to Testing	Cancelled Tests
Pre-employment	122	121	1	1	0	1	0	0	0
Random	1,430	1,428	2	2	1	1	0	0	0
Post-Accident	454	454	0	0	0	0	0	0	0
Reasonable Suspicion	18	7	11	11	1	9	0	0	0
Return-to-Duty	23	23	0	0	0	0	0	0	0
Follow-up	286	286	0	0	0	0	0	0	0
TOTAL	**2,333**	**2,319**	**14**	**14**	**2**	**11**	**0**	**0**	**0**

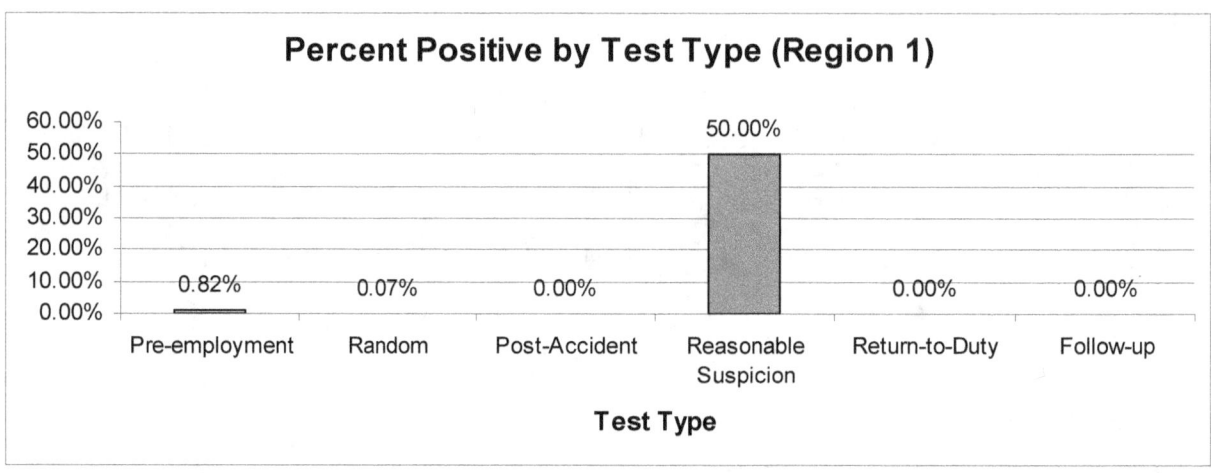

Figure 57. Percent Positive for All Employee Categories by Test Type for Region 1

60

4.5.2 Alcohol Test Results for Region 2

Table 58 provides alcohol test results for all employee categories by test type within Region 2. Figure 58 illustrates the percent positive for all employee categories by test type within Region 2.

Table 58. Alcohol Results for All Employee Categories by Test Type for Region 2

Test Type	Total Number of Screening Test Results	Screening Tests with Results Below 0.02	Screening Tests with Results 0.02 or Greater	Number of Confirmation Test Results	Confirmation Tests with Results 0.02 to 0.039	Confirmation Tests with Results 0.04 or Greater	"Shy Lung" with No Medical Explanation	Other Refusals to Submit to Testing	Cancelled Tests
Pre-employment	1,741	1,740	1	1	0	1	0	0	0
Random	8,325	8,304	19	19	7	11	2	0	5
Post-Accident	2,314	2,309	4	4	0	3	1	0	0
Reasonable Suspicion	52	38	14	14	4	9	0	0	0
Return-to-Duty	56	56	0	0	0	0	0	0	0
Follow-up	1,663	1,656	7	7	3	3	0	0	0
TOTAL	**14,151**	**14,103**	**45**	**45**	**14**	**27**	**3**	**0**	**5**

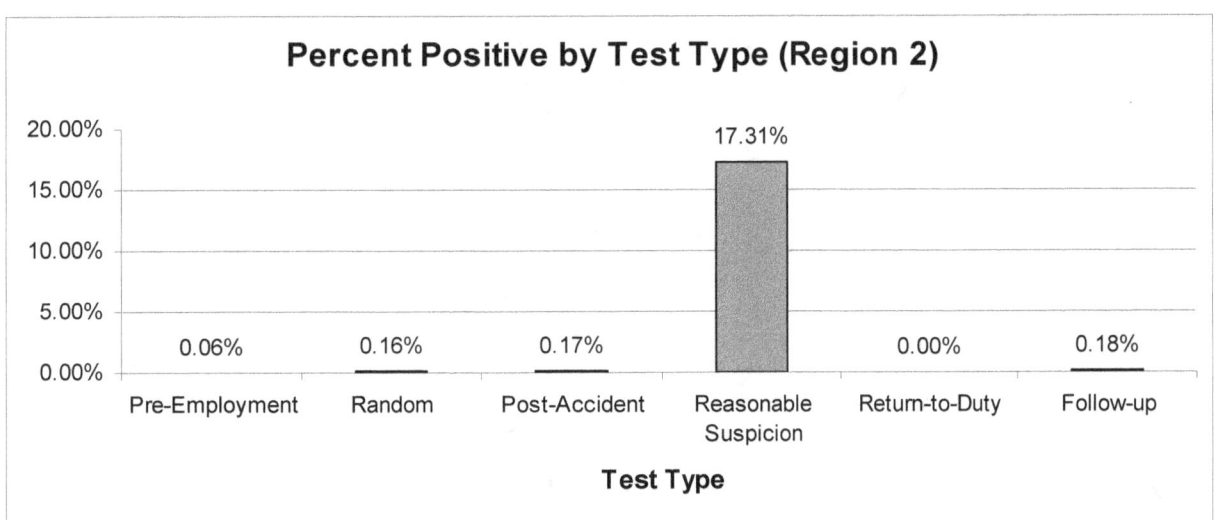

Figure 58. Percent Positive for All Employee Categories by Test Type for Region 2

61

4.5.3 Alcohol Test Results for Region 3

Table 59 provides alcohol test results for all employee categories by test type within Region 3. Figure 59 illustrates the percent positive for all employee categories by test type within Region 3.

Table 59. Alcohol Results for All Employee Categories by Test Type for Region 3

Test Type	Total Number of Screening Test Results	Screening Tests with Results Below 0.02	Screening Tests with Results 0.02 or Greater	Number of Confirmation Test Results	Confirmation Tests with Results 0.02 to 0.039	Confirmation Tests with Results 0.04 or Greater	"Shy Lung" with No Medical Explanation	Other Refusals to Submit to Testing	Cancelled Tests
Pre-employment	4,019	4,012	7	7	0	6	0	0	0
Random	5,939	5,925	13	12	2	7	0	1	2
Post-Accident	1,077	1,075	2	2	0	2	0	0	0
Reasonable Suspicion	97	77	18	18	5	12	1	1	0
Return-to-Duty	116	116	0	0	0	0	0	0	0
Follow-up	1,032	1,026	6	6	3	3	0	0	0
TOTAL	**12,280**	**12,231**	**46**	**45**	**10**	**30**	**1**	**2**	**2**

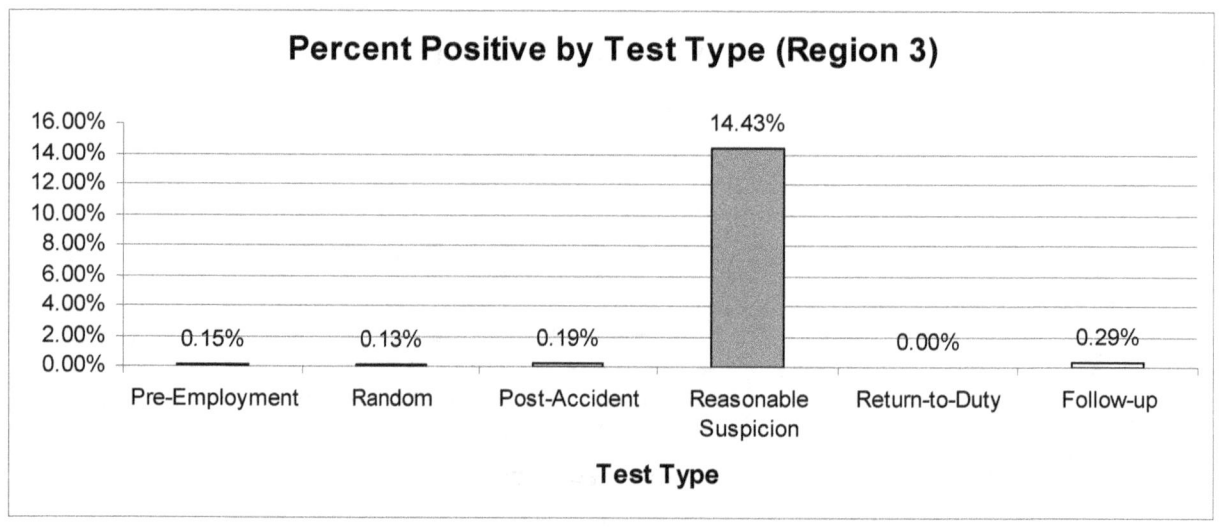

Figure 59. Percent Positive for All Employee Categories by Test Type for Region 3

4.5.4 Alcohol Test Results for Region 4

Table 60 provides alcohol test results for all employee categories by test type within Region 4. Figure 60 illustrates the percent positive for all employee categories by test type within Region 4.

Table 60. Alcohol Results for All Employee Categories by Test Type for Region 4

Test Type	Total Number of Screening Test Results	Screening Tests with Results Below 0.02	Screening Tests with Results 0.02 or Greater	Number of Confirmation Test Results	Confirmation Tests with Results 0.02 to 0.039	Confirmation Tests with Results 0.04 or Greater	"Shy Lung" with No Medical Explanation	Other Refusals to Submit to Testing	Cancelled Tests
Pre-employment	1,620	1,610	10	2	0	1	0	0	0
Random	4,798	4,791	6	4	1	1	1	0	1
Post-Accident	1,694	1,691	2	1	0	1	0	1	1
Reasonable Suspicion	48	38	7	7	1	6	0	3	2
Return-to-Duty	48	48	0	0	0	0	0	0	0
Follow-up	215	212	3	3	0	1	0	0	0
TOTAL	**8,423**	**8,390**	**28**	**17**	**2**	**10**	**1**	**4**	**4**

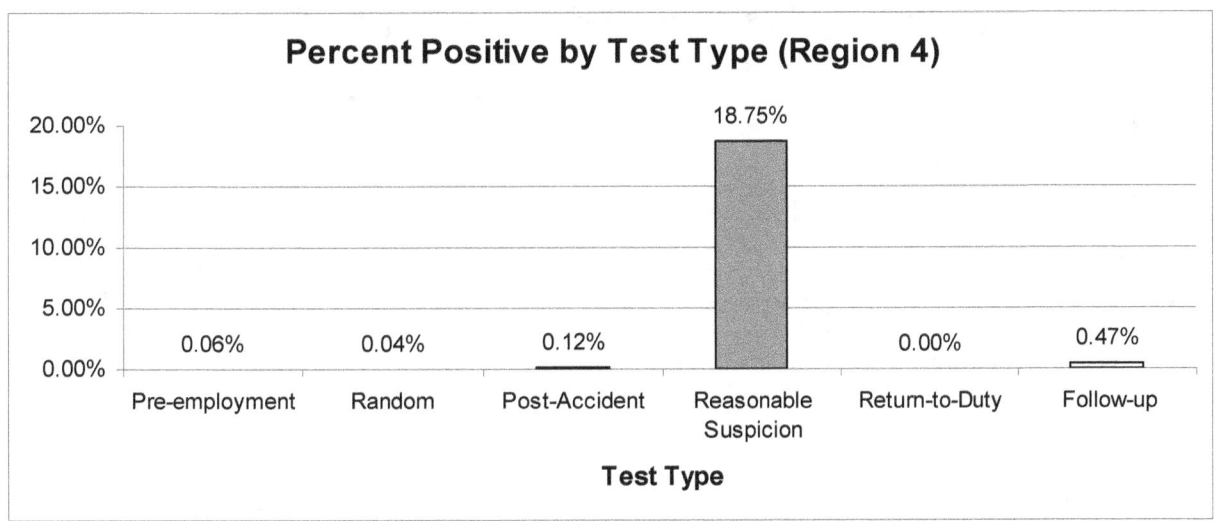

Figure 60. Percent Positive for All Employee Categories by Test Type for Region 4

63

4.5.5 Alcohol Test Results for Region 5

Table 61 provides alcohol test results for all employee categories by test type within Region 5. Figure 61 illustrates the percent positive for all employee categories by test type within Region 5.

Table 61. Alcohol Results for All Employee Categories by Test Type for Region 5

Test Type	Total Number of Screening Test Results	Screening Tests with Results Below 0.02	Screening Tests with Results 0.02 or Greater	Number of Confirmation Test Results	Confirmation Tests with Results 0.02 to 0.039	Confirmation Tests with Results 0.04 or Greater	"Shy Lung" with No Medical Explanation	Other Refusals to Submit to Testing	Cancelled Tests
Pre-employment	2,020	2,017	3	3	0	2	0	0	0
Random	5,125	5,107	14	14	5	9	2	2	13
Post-Accident	2,283	2,276	6	6	4	2	0	1	0
Reasonable Suspicion	114	95	18	18	4	13	0	1	0
Return-to-Duty	86	85	1	1	0	1	0	0	0
Follow-up	480	474	6	6	1	4	0	0	0
TOTAL	**10,108**	**10,054**	**48**	**48**	**14**	**31**	**2**	**4**	**13**

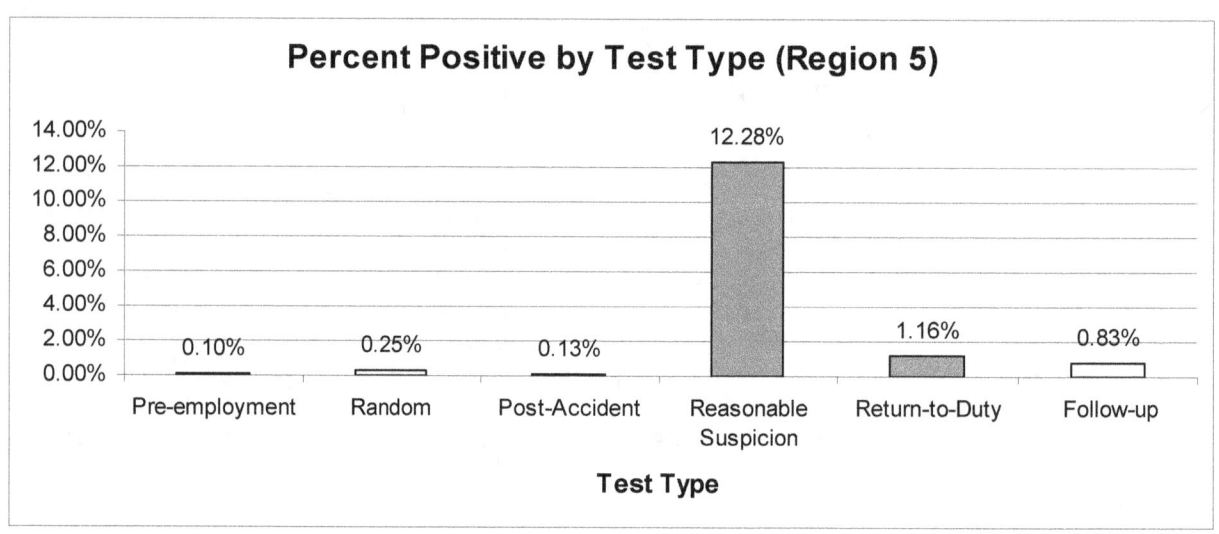

Figure 61. Percent Positive for All Employee Categories by Test Type for Region 5

4.5.6 Alcohol Test Results for Region 6

Table 62 provides alcohol test results for all employee categories by test type within Region 6. Figure 62 illustrates the percent positive for all employee categories by test type within Region 6.

Table 62. Alcohol Results for All Employee Categories by Test Type for Region 6

Test Type	Total Number of Screening Test Results	Screening Tests with Results Below 0.02	Screening Tests with Results 0.02 or Greater	Number of Confirmation Test Results	Confirmation Tests with Results 0.02 to 0.039	Confirmation Tests with Results 0.04 or Greater	"Shy Lung" with No Medical Explanation	Other Refusals to Submit to Testing	Cancelled Tests
Pre-employment	892	891	1	1	1	0	0	0	1
Random	2,714	2,709	5	5	1	3	0	0	2
Post-Accident	899	896	2	2	1	1	0	1	0
Reasonable Suspicion	32	20	12	12	3	9	0	0	0
Return-to-Duty	14	14	0	0	0	0	0	0	0
Follow-up	100	98	2	2	2	0	0	0	0
TOTAL	**4,651**	**4,628**	**22**	**22**	**8**	**13**	**0**	**1**	**3**

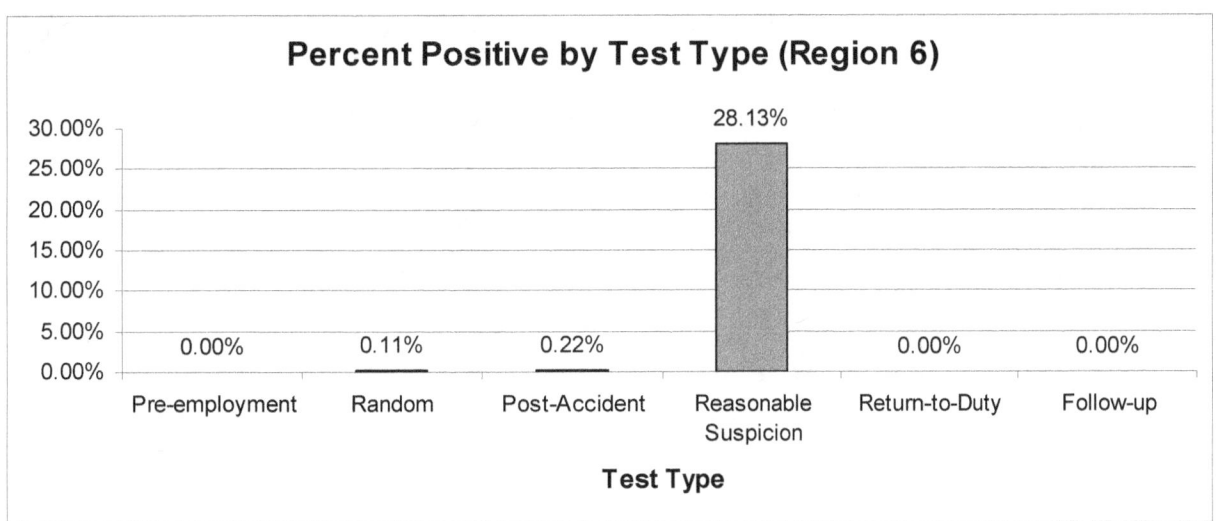

Figure 62. Percent Positive for All Employee Categories by Test Type for Region 6

4.5.7 Alcohol Test Results for Region 7

Table 63 provides alcohol test results for all employee categories by test type within Region 7. Figure 63 illustrates the percent positive for all employee categories by test type within Region 7.

Table 63. Alcohol Results for All Employee Categories by Test Type for Region 7

Test Type	Total Number of Screening Test Results	Screening Tests with Results Below 0.02	Screening Tests with Results 0.02 or Greater	Number of Confirmation Test Results	Confirmation Tests with Results 0.02 to 0.039	Confirmation Tests with Results 0.04 or Greater	"Shy Lung" with No Medical Explanation	Other Refusals to Submit to Testing	Cancelled Tests
Pre-employment	166	165	1	1	0	0	0	0	0
Random	1,250	1,244	4	4	3	1	1	1	2
Post-Accident	387	387	0	0	0	0	0	0	0
Reasonable Suspicion	13	9	4	4	0	4	0	0	0
Return-to-Duty	24	24	0	0	0	0	0	0	0
Follow-up	42	42	0	0	0	0	0	0	0
TOTAL	**1,882**	**1,871**	**9**	**9**	**3**	**5**	**1**	**1**	**2**

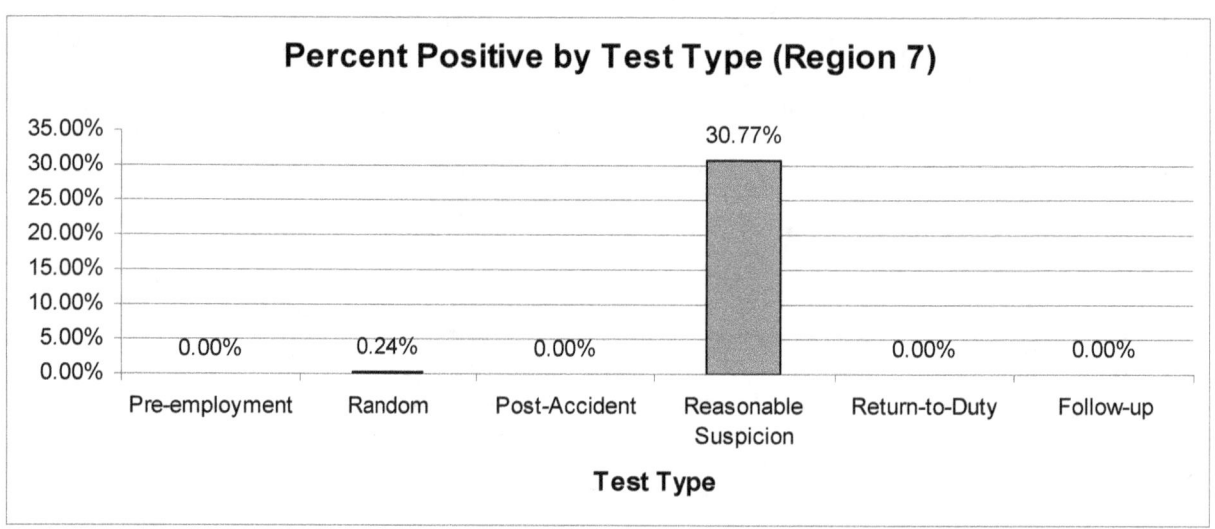

Figure 63. Percent Positive for All Employee Categories by Test Type for Region 7

4.5.8 Alcohol Test Results for Region 8

Table 64 provides alcohol test results for all employee categories by test type within Region 8. Figure 64 illustrates the percent positive for all employee categories by test type within Region 8.

Table 64. Alcohol Results for All Employee Categories by Test Type for Region 8

Test Type	Total Number of Screening Test Results	Screening Tests with Results Below 0.02	Screening Tests with Results 0.02 or Greater	Number of Confirmation Test Results	Confirmation Tests with Results 0.02 to 0.039	Confirmation Tests with Results 0.04 or Greater	"Shy Lung" with No Medical Explanation	Other Refusals to Submit to Testing	Cancelled Tests
Pre-employment	88	88	0	0	0	0	0	0	0
Random	1,101	1,083	17	4	0	2	0	1	0
Post-Accident	235	235	0	0	0	0	0	0	0
Reasonable Suspicion	21	12	8	8	3	4	0	1	0
Return-to-Duty	4	4	0	0	0	0	0	0	0
Follow-up	61	61	0	0	0	0	0	0	0
TOTAL	**1,510**	**1,483**	**25**	**12**	**3**	**6**	**0**	**2**	**0**

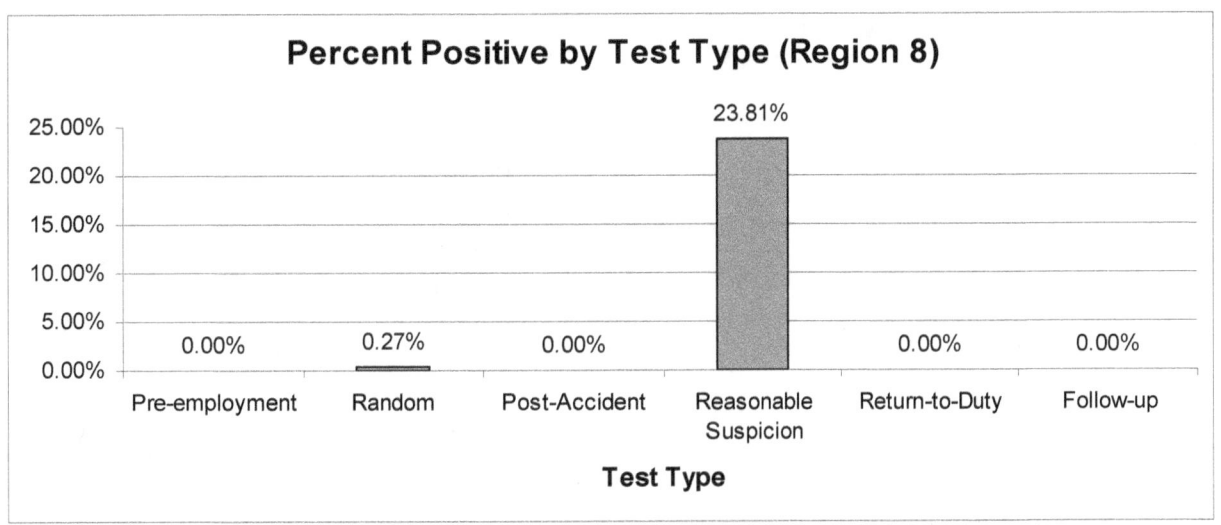

Figure 64. Percent Positive for All Employee Categories by Test Type for Region 8

4.5.9 Alcohol Test Results for Region 9

Table 65 provides alcohol test results for all employee categories by test type within Region 9. Figure 65 illustrates the percent positive for all employee categories by test type within Region 9.

Table 65. Alcohol Results for All Employee Categories by Test Type for Region 9

Test Type	Total Number of Screening Test Results	Screening Tests with Results Below 0.02	Screening Tests with Results 0.02 or Greater	Number of Confirmation Test Results	Confirmation Tests with Results 0.02 to 0.039	Confirmation Tests with Results 0.04 or Greater	"Shy Lung" with No Medical Explanation	Other Refusals to Submit to Testing	Cancelled Tests
Pre-employment	2,524	2,520	4	4	2	1	0	0	1
Random	5,956	5,940	13	14	6	8	2	1	4
Post-Accident	2,376	2,371	5	5	2	3	0	0	0
Reasonable Suspicion	86	58	27	25	5	17	0	1	0
Return-to-Duty	80	80	0	0	0	0	0	0	0
Follow-up	1,145	1,144	0	0	0	0	0	1	3
TOTAL	**12,167**	**12,113**	**49**	**48**	**15**	**29**	**2**	**3**	**8**

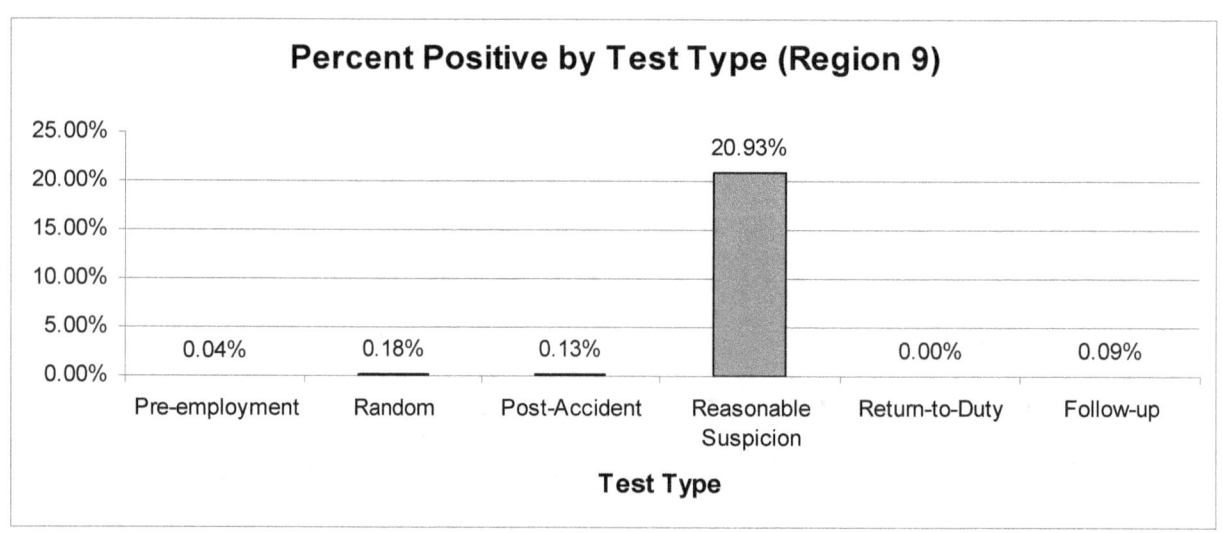

Figure 65. Percent Positive for All Employee Categories by Test Type for Region 9

4.5.10 Alcohol Test Results for Region 10

Table 66 provides alcohol test results for all employee categories by test type within Region 10. Figure 66 illustrates the percent positive for all employee categories by test type within Region 10.

Table 66. Alcohol Results for All Employee Categories by Test Type for Region 10

Test Type	Total Number of Screening Test Results	Screening Tests with Results Below 0.02	Screening Tests with Results 0.02 or Greater	Number of Confirmation Test Results	Confirmation Tests with Results 0.02 to 0.039	Confirmation Tests with Results 0.04 or Greater	"Shy Lung" with No Medical Explanation	Other Refusals to Submit to Testing	Cancelled Tests
Pre-employment	253	253	0	0	0	0	0	0	0
Random	1,838	1,835	2	2	2	0	1	0	2
Post-Accident	527	527	0	0	0	0	0	0	2
Reasonable Suspicion	20	15	5	5	1	4	0	0	0
Return-to-Duty	6	6	0	0	0	0	0	0	0
Follow-up	82	82	0	0	0	0	0	0	0
TOTAL	**2,726**	**2,718**	**7**	**7**	**3**	**4**	**1**	**0**	**4**

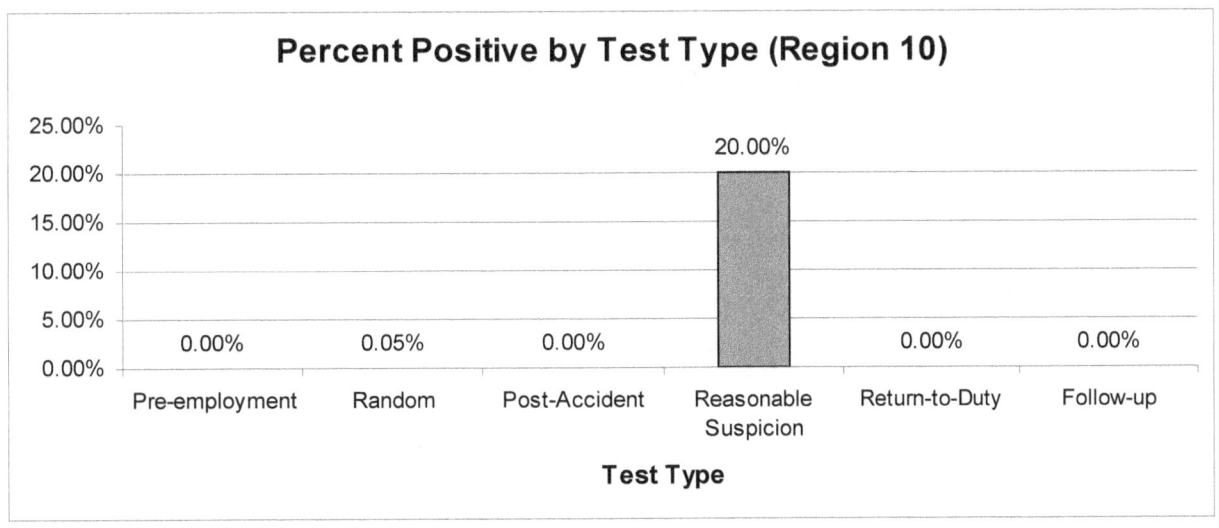

Figure 66. Percent Positive for All Employee Categories by Test Type for Region 10

Appendix A. MIS Data Collection Form

U.S. DEPARTMENT OF TRANSPORTATION DRUG AND ALCOHOL TESTING MIS DATA COLLECTION FORM

Calendar Year Covered by this Report: _____

OMB No 2105-0529

I. Employer:

Company Name:_____

Doing Business As (DBA) Name (if applicable):_____

Address:_____ E-mail: _____

Name of Certifying Official: _____ Signature: _____

Telephone: (____)_____ Date Certified: _____

Prepared by (if different): _____ Telephone: (____)_____

C/TPA Name and Telephone (if applicable): _____ (____)_____

Check the DOT agency for which you are reporting MIS data; and complete the information on that same line as appropriate:

___ FMCSA – Motor Carrier: DOT #: _____ Owner-operator: (circle one) YES or NO Exempt (Circle One) YES or NO

___ FAA – Aviation: Certificate # (if applicable): _____ Plan / Registration # (if applicable):_____

___ RSPA – Pipeline: (Check) Gas Gathering__ Gas Transmission__ Gas Distribution__ Transport Hazardous Liquids__ Transport Carbon Dioxide__

___ FRA – Railroad: Total Number of observed/documented Part 219 "Rule G" Observations for covered employees: _____

___ USCG – Maritime: Vessel ID # (USCG- or State-Issued): _____ (If more than one vessel, list separately.)

___ FTA – Transit

II. Covered Employees: (A) Enter Total Number Safety-Sensitive Employees In All Employee Categories: [   ]

(B) Enter Total Number of Employee Categories: [   ]

(C)

Employee Category	Total Number of Employees in this Category	If you have multiple employee categories, complete Sections I and II (A) & (B). Take that filled-in form and make one copy for each employee category and complete Sections II (C), III, and IV for each separate employee category.

III. Drug Testing Data:

Type of Test	1 Total Number Of Test Results [Should equal the sum of Columns 2, 3, 9, 10, 11, and 12]	2 Verified Negative Results	3 Verified Positive Results ~ For One Or More Drugs	4 Positive For Marijuana	5 Positive For Cocaine	6 Positive For PCP	7 Positive For Opiates	8 Positive For Amphetamines	9 Refusal Results — Adulterated	10 Refusal Results — Substituted	11 Refusal Results — "Shy Bladder" With No Medical Explanation	12 Refusal Results — Other Refusals To Submit To Testing	13 Cancelled Results
Pre-Employment													
Random													
Post-Accident													
Reasonable Susp./Cause													
Return-to-Duty													
Follow-Up													
TOTAL													

IV. Alcohol Testing Data:

Type of Test	1 Total Number Of Screening Test Results [Should equal the sum of Columns 2, 3, 7, and 8]	2 Screening Tests With Results Below 0.02	3 Screening Tests With Results 0.02 Or Greater	4 Number Of Confirmation Tests Results	5 Confirmation Tests With Results 0.02 Through 0.039	6 Confirmation Tests With Results 0.04 Or Greater	7 Refusal Results — "Shy Lung" ~ With No Medical Explanation	8 Refusal Results — Other Refusals To Submit To Testing	9 Cancelled Results
Pre-Employment									
Random									
Post-Accident									
Reasonable Susp./Cause									
Return-to-Duty									
Follow-Up									
TOTAL									

Appendix B. Contact Information

For additional information regarding the FTA's drug and alcohol testing requirements, please contact the following individuals:

Jerry Powers
Drug and Alcohol Program Manager
Office of Safety and Security
Federal Transit Administration
Volpe National Transportation Systems Center
55 Broadway
Cambridge, MA 02142
Gerald.Powers@dot.gov

Mike Redington
Program Manager/Transportation Industry Analyst
Volpe National Transportation Systems Center
55 Broadway
Cambridge, MA 02142
Michael.Redington@dot.gov

Eve Rutyna
Transportation Industry Analyst
Volpe National Transportation Systems Center
55 Broadway
Cambridge, MA 02142
Eve.Rutyna@dot.gov

For assistance in accessing the FTA Office of Safety and Security Web site and using the Internet reporting system, contact the FTA DAMIS Project Office at (617) 494-6336 or via e-mail at FTA.damis@volpe.dot.gov. Contact the FTA Safety and Security Clearinghouse at (617) 494-2116 for additional copies of this report as well as technical assistance materials, including the *Implementation Guidelines for Drug and Alcohol Regulations in Mass Transit* and *Best Practices Manual: FTA Drug and Alcohol Testing Program*. Documents can also be obtained from the FTA Safety and Security Clearinghouse Web site at: http://transit-safety.volpe.dot.gov/publications/order/default.asp. You may also send e-mail directly to FTA.clearinghouse@volpe.dot.gov.

Appendix C. Glossary of Terms

Accident: An occurrence associated with the operation of a vehicle, if as a result:
(1) An individual dies.
(2) An individual suffers a bodily injury and immediately receives medical treatment away from the scene of the accident.
(3) With respect to an occurrence in which the mass transit vehicle involved is a bus, electric bus, van, or automobile, one or more vehicles incurs disabling damage and is transported away from the scene by a tow truck or other vehicle.
(4) With respect to an occurrence in which the mass transit vehicle involved is a rail car, trolley car, trolley bus, or vessel, the mass transit vehicle is removed from revenue service.

Alcohol Concentration: The alcohol in a volume of breath, expressed in terms of grams of alcohol per 210 liters of breath as indicated by a breath test.

Amphetamines: Includes racemic, amphetamine, extroamphetamine, and methamphetamine. These are potent stimulants that can be swallowed, snorted, or injected. They reduce the desire to sleep or eat and can induce a sense of aroused euphoria, accompanied by feelings of increased power, strength, energy, self-assertion, focus, and motivation. Because the body does not readily break down amphetamines, these feelings, which are often intense and ephemeral, may last several hours. Severe mental depression and fatigue can set in when the euphoric feelings wear off.

Armed Security Personnel: Employees who provide security and carry a firearm.

Canceled or Invalid Test: In drug testing, a drug test that has been declared invalid by a Medical Review Officer (MRO). In alcohol testing, a test that is deemed to be invalid. It is neither a positive nor a negative test.

CDL/Non-Revenue Vehicle: Job category including any transit employee who holds a Commercial Driver's License (CDL), performs a function requiring a CDL, and is not included in any other job category.

Cocaine: An addictive substance that comes from coca leaves or is made synthetically. It appears as a white powder that is snorted, ingested, injected, freebased (smoked), or applied directly to the nasal membrane or gums. Cocaine acts as a stimulant to the central nervous system. It gives the user a feeling of exhilaration. The chemicals in cocaine trick the brain into feeling it has experienced pleasure when in fact it has not.

Confirmation (or Confirmatory) Test: In drug testing, a second analytical procedure to identify the presence of a specific drug or metabolite that is independent of the screening test and that uses a different technique and chemical principle from those of the screening test in order to ensure reliability and accuracy. In alcohol testing, a second test following a screening test with a result of 0.02 or greater that provides quantitative data of alcohol concentration.

Consortium: An entity, such as a group or association of employers, operators, recipients, subrecipients, or contractors, that provides drug testing services and acts on behalf of the employer.

Contractor: A person or organization that provides a service for a recipient, subrecipient, employer, or operator consistent with a specific understanding or arrangement. The understanding can be a written contract or an informal arrangement that reflects an ongoing relationship between the parties.

Covered Employee: A person, such as an applicant, transferee, or volunteer who perform a safety-sensitive function for a recipient, subrecipient, employer, or operator.

Drug Metabolite: The specific substance produced when the human body metabolizes a given prohibited drug as it passes through and is excreted in urine.

Drug Test: The laboratory analysis of a urine specimen collected in accordance with 49 CFR Part 40 and analyzed in a Department of Health and Human Services (DHHS)-approved laboratory.

Education: Efforts that include the display and distribution of informational materials, a community service hotline telephone number for employee assistance, and the transit entity policy regarding drug use and alcohol misuse in the workplace.

Employee: An individual designated in a Department of Transportation (DOT) agency regulation as subject to drug and/or alcohol testing; includes applicants for employment.

Employer: A recipient or other entity that provides mass transportation services or performs a safety-sensitive function for such recipient or other entity. This term includes subrecipients, operators, and contractors.

Follow-up Testing: Drug or alcohol test that is required for an employee who is returned to safety-sensitive duty. The employee is subject to at least six unannounced tests for at least 12 months after returning to duty. The exact number and frequency of tests is prescribed by the Substance Abuse Professional (SAP), who may order tests for up to 60 months after return to duty. The SAP often requires the employee to submit to both a drug and an alcohol test even if only one of the tests was at issue. Follow-up testing is separate from and in addition to random testing. Part 655 incorporates follow-up testing under return-to-duty testing (i.e., return to duty/follow-up testing) as one of five required FTA tests. It was previously listed separately as one of six required FTA tests.

Marijuana: Derived from the hemp plant, it comes in a variety of colors such as green, brown, and a gray mixture of leaves. THC (delta-9-tetrahydrocannabinol) is the primary active chemical in marijuana. It is absorbed quickly into fatty tissues and stored for a long time. The potency and strength of the chemical causes people to use the drug for the mildly tranquilizing, mood- and perception-altering effects it produces. The test for marijuana also includes its metabolites.

Opiates: Known as narcotic analgesics, includes heroin, morphine, and codeine. Opiates are derived from a sap taken from a seedpod of the plant, *papaver somniferum* (or poppy plant). General effects include sedation, slowed reflexes, raspy speech, sluggish movements, slowed breathing, cold skin, and vomiting. The synthetic form of opiates, known as a designer drug, is even more deadly and addictive.

Phencyclidine (PCP): Originally developed as an anesthetic; has adverse side effects that limit its medical use to a tranquilizer for large animals. In people, PCP acts as both a depressant and a hallucinogen and sometimes as a stimulant. PCP can cause distorted bodily perceptions and a feeling of disassociation in which the mind feels separated from the body. These effects can be very upsetting to some people, who may panic as a result.

Positive Rate: The sum of the annual number of verified positive results for random drug tests conducted under 49 CFR Part 655 plus the annual number of refusals to submit to a random drug test, divided by the total number of test results.

Post-Accident Testing: Tests required following an accident involving a fatality or following an accident that meets any of three other criteria if the employee's involvement cannot be completely discounted as a contributing factor: (1) a person suffers a bodily injury and immediately receives medical attention from the scene, (2) when any vehicle involved in the accident incurs damage requiring it to be transported away from the scene by a tow truck or other vehicle, or (3) the mass transit vehicle involved is a rail car, trolley car, trolley bus, or vessel and is removed from revenue service due to the accident.

Pre-employment Testing: Testing of candidates (including existing non-safety-sensitive employees and applicants for employment) for a safety-sensitive position and of employees who have not performed a safety-sensitive function for more than 90 consecutive calendar days, regardless of the reason, and have been removed from the employer's random selection pool during that time.

A negative pre-employment test for drugs is required by FTA as a condition for performing safety-sensitive duties under these circumstances. Pre-employment alcohol tests are not required but are permitted under Part 655, providing that they are performed in accordance with the testing procedures in Part 40. The alcohol tests are included in the data presented in Chapter 4 of this report because they are conducted per DOT standards and are required by many employers. The Omnibus Testing Act required a negative pre-employment alcohol test, but FTA suspended the requirement on May 10, 1995, as the result of a U.S. Court of Appeals decision. FTA decided to allow but not require pre-employment alcohol testing in Part 655.

Random Testing: Considered by FTA to be the most effective deterrent to drug use and alcohol misuse as well as the most reliable indicator of drug use and alcohol misuse within an employer and in the industry as a whole, provided it is unannounced and unpredictable. Selections for testing must be based on a scientifically valid random-number selection method, to ensure that all safety-sensitive employees have an equal chance of being selected for testing.

Random Testing Rate: The number of drug tests equal to at least 50 percent of the total number of safety-sensitive employees and, of alcohol tests equal to at least 10 percent of the total number of safety-sensitive employees must be conducted each year by this method.

Reasonable Suspicion Testing: Required when an employer has reasonable suspicion that an employee has used a prohibited drug or has misused alcohol as defined in the regulations. Must be based on specific, contemporaneous, articulable observations made by a trained supervisor concerning the appearance, behavior, speech, or body odor of a safety-sensitive employee.

Recipient: An entity receiving federal financial assistance under Section 5307, 5309, or 5311 of the Federal Transit Act or under Sections 103(e)(4) of Title 23 of the U.S. Code.

Refusal to Submit (to an alcohol test): When a covered employee fails to provide adequate breath for testing without a valid medical explanation.

Refusal to Submit (to a drug test): When a covered employee fails to provide a urine sample as required by 49 CFR Part 40 without a valid medical explanation after receiving notice of the requirement to be tested, or engages in conduct that clearly obstructs the testing process.

Return-to-Duty Testing: Drug and/or alcohol test that is required for a safety-sensitive employee who completes a course of treatment prescribed by a SAP after testing positive for drugs or alcohol or refusing to submit to a required test. A negative result for the type (drug or alcohol) of positive or refused test is required before the employee can be returned to duty. SAPs often require the employee to submit to both a drug and an alcohol test even if only one of the tests was at issue.

Revenue Vehicle Control/Dispatch: Includes employees who control the movement of revenue service vehicles. The key consideration is the type of work performed rather than a particular job title. FTA decided not to attempt a universal definition of "dispatchers" in Part 655. Instead, each employer determines whether its particular dispatcher performs or may perform a safety-sensitive function.

Revenue Vehicle and Equipment Maintenance: Includes employees who maintain revenue service vehicles or equipment, as well as many maintenance contract employees who perform routine, ongoing repair or maintenance for FTA recipients and subrecipients that have employees, including supervisors, who perform or could be called upon to perform any of the FTA safety-sensitive functions. Maintenance contractors of 5311 funding recipients are not subject to the testing regulations. Additionally, recipients that operate in areas with a population of 200,000 or less and contract out maintenance services are no longer required to comply.

Revenue Vehicle Operation: Safety-sensitive job category; includes employees who operate a revenue service vehicle, regardless of whether it is in service.

Safety-Sensitive Function: Any of the following duties:

- Operating a revenue service vehicle, including when not in revenue service

- Operating a non-revenue service vehicle that is required to be operated by the holder of a CDL
- Controlling dispatch or movement of a revenue service vehicle
- Maintaining a revenue service vehicle or equipment used in revenue service, unless the recipient receives Section 5311 funding and contracts out such services
- Providing security and carrying a firearm

Screening Test (or Initial Test): In drug testing, an immunoassay screen to eliminate negative urine specimens from further analysis. In alcohol testing, an analytical procedure to determine whether an employee may have a prohibited concentration of alcohol in a breath specimen.

Transit System: The public entity that receives the federal grant (direct grant recipient), whether or not that recipient provides mass transit services directly.

Vehicle and Equipment Maintenance: Function including any person repairing or maintaining revenue service vehicles or other equipment used in revenue service.

Violation Rate: Refers to the sum of the annual number of results from random alcohol tests conducted under 49 CFR Part 655 that have alcohol concentrations of 0.04 or greater plus the annual number of refusals to submit to alcohol tests, divided by the sum of the annual number of random alcohol tests conducted plus the annual number of refusals to submit to a drug test.

Verified Negative (drug test result): A drug test result reviewed by an MRO and determined to have no evidence of prohibited drug use.

Verified Positive (drug test result): A drug test result reviewed by an MRO and determined to have evidence of prohibited drug use.